Boundless

Annette —
I am so grateful for your
work and your role in bringing
our daughter into the world.
With love,
Chrissy

BOUNDLESS

An Abortion Doctor
Becomes a Mother

Christine Henneberg

979-8-9860667-0-7 Paperback
979-8-9860667-1-4 Ebook

Library of Congress Control Number: 2022907949
Printed in San Francisco, CA

Lyric reprint rights are as follows:

(Sittin' On) The Dock Of The Bay
Words and Music by Steve Cropper and Otis Redding
Copyright (c) 1968 IRVING MUSIC, INC.
Copyright Renewed
All Rights Reserved Used by Permission
Reprinted by Permission of Hal Leonard LLC

The Sound Of Music
Lyrics by Oscar Hammerstein II
Music by Richard Rodgers
Copyright (c) 1959 Williamson Music Company c/o Concord Music Publishing
Copyright Renewed
All Rights Reserved Used by Permission
Reprinted by Permission of Hal Leonard LLC

In this book, all names are pseudonyms other than those of my family, friends, and a few physician colleagues. The names and some identifying details of patients have been changed in order to protect their privacy.

Cover and interior design by Sarah Lahay

For my daughter.

FOREWORD

I WROTE *BOUNDLESS* IN 2018, from a time and place of great privilege. In addition to being a white upper-middle-class American, as a woman and a doctor I have always known the privilege of geography—a privilege that over the past three years has become increasingly, tragically evident. I live and work in California, where abortion is (for the time being) legal until twenty-four weeks, and covered by public health insurance. This is in contrast to large swaths of the United States, where, despite *Roe v. Wade*'s protections, accessible, affordable abortion has never been a reality.

Since I wrote *Boundless*, new state abortion restrictions and outright challenges to *Roe* have come at an alarming rate. In September of 2021, the state of Texas banned all abortions after roughly six weeks, a decision that has been thus far upheld by the U.S. Supreme Court. As I write this, the overturning of *Roe* in 2022 feels almost certain—a development that will leave vast "abortion deserts" throughout much of America.

A thought that often crosses my mind these days when I perform an abortion—particularly when the woman is a teenager, or homeless, or a victim of intimate partner violence—is: *what if she were in Texas?* In other words: what if she couldn't have this procedure today? I try to imagine what would come next for her. Would she find some other way? Order pills from the internet? Travel across state lines? In many cases I know the answer is: *for this woman, there would be no other way. She simply does not have the money, or the stability, or the privacy to make any of those solutions work.* If she were in Texas, she would be forced to have this baby.

For readers in 2022, this question will throw a dark shadow over many of the stories and the women in this book: *what if she were in Texas?* It makes for a chilling, sometime devastating thought exercise—although that wasn't my original intention. I did not write *Boundless* as a warning about the threat to abortion rights—even though I am a staunch supporter of those rights. Nor did I aim to simply collect a handful of stories about the women whose abortions I have performed.

A doctor (and any writer) who tells true stories must always ask herself to whom those stories belong. I believe that each woman's abortion story belongs to her, and her alone. Those stories—what happened to her, and why, and what meaning it had in her life—are not mine to tell. Instead, what I tell here is my story: the story of what it felt like to care for those women, and what I learned from the experience of being their doctor.

As for the stories about family—my own and others: I do not intend to give an objective or balanced account of events or what they meant to each of the individuals involved. Rather, I recount my experience of observing and in some cases living through these events. I intend to show how they shaped me and pushed me to expand my own boundaries.

Boundless is the story of how I learned *what motherhood is*—its choices, sacrifices, hopes, joys, and regrets—through my training and practice as an abortion doctor. It is my hope that this story can wedge into a very tiny space in the American abortion conversation, a space where supporters of abortion rights can fully acknowledge, respect, and even love the lives that are, for any reason, conceived but not born. What would happen to the conversation if we opened that space, met one another there, and stayed for a while? It is not a comfortable space to dwell, but I believe it is an important one. It is the space where I live and work every day. It is, indeed, an extraordinary privilege.

May 31 2022

PROLOGUE

AN IMAGE IN BLACK and white: boundaries created by contrast.

In an unseen, untouchable place, sound waves penetrate fluid thicker than water, undulating at a low frequency until they bump into something—calcified calvarium, black bladder, a spiraled and sinewy cord that pulses in the darkness—then bounce back, reversing course at varied wavelengths to form the image on my screen.

This *chiaroscuro*, a blur to the untrained eye, is as familiar and interpretable to me now as the stone steps that curve through my garden in the dark, under the soles of my bare feet. What I call it, what words I choose to describe it to the person who lies on the table, bare and vulnerable, depends on forces more powerful and

1

penetrating than any ultrasound wave. If I am unsure, I can always fall back on the safest word, the word that may be clinical and unfeeling but is at least always accurate: pregnancy.

This is the word I use when her face is turned toward the wall, when she doesn't want to know the details of what I've found—only whether I can help her. "Yes, I see the pregnancy. It'll be fine. We can do it today."

And this is the word I use for an entirely different conversation, one that begins with, "Yes, I see it. Wonderful. Shall I show you?" She looks up at me, beaming, and I swivel the screen toward her and point out what I see:

The window created by the probe is crescent-shaped, like a flashlight beam in a cartoon. Inside that beam, the dense, muscular uterus appears as a large gray oval. "Here is the uterus, do you see? Inside of that, you see the fluid that holds the pregnancy—it looks black on the screen. This is called the gestational sac. Inside that sac is a white ring, like a halo, called the yolk sac. Right here. This is the early nutritional source to the pregnancy. And there—do you see? That little white bean shape next to it? That's the embryo. I'm measuring it now. It's about six weeks in size. That flicker—do you see it? That's the heartbeat. Yes! Congratulations."

I am a new doctor, just six months out of training. These are the skills that I can fall back on: black and white. Choice of words. Knowing what to say and when. Different circumstances call for different explanations, and I know how to draw the boundaries and keep things in their separate compartments where they belong. Or at least I think I do. But I am beginning to sense that things may not be as clear as they first appeared. Like an ultrasound image warped and shot with shadows, dials that refuse to pull things into focus, the tools I once relied on have recently, more frequently, begun to fail me. It is as though a black-and-white image, flattened into two dimensions, is no longer adequate for the truths I need to capture, the stories I have to tell.

In the six months following my graduation from residency, I slept as though my life depended on it. At the graduation party in July, I drank two glasses of wine, danced for half an hour, and asked Mo to drive me home before midnight. I fell asleep in the car.

Mo and I went to Barcelona for the month of August. I slept on the plane, the train, a bench in the lobby of a Catalan art museum. Returning home in September, we bought a house; I slept in every room including the bathroom and the kitchen. At night I slept fourteen hours at a stretch, ravenous when I woke at midday. We hung a hammock in the backyard and for a week I slept in it every afternoon, stirring to the pale light of dusk and the hum of Mo's car in the driveway.

But that's over now. It is dark, before dawn, the Earth turning toward winter. I'm back in the habit of rising early. It is as though my mind remembers that this is the hour for history-taking, investigation, examination. I don't mind it. I like slipping out of bed before Mo is awake, before the birds begin their chatter, before the Northern California sun peers over the fence onto the yard: the potted lemon tree, the unruly lavender. It's early December, our first winter in this house, and my first writing in this office, a converted garden shed at the end of a stone path in our backyard. I am at my desk in sweats and slippers, my legs wrapped under an old down comforter, next to a space heater that hums like an insect and warms my left side but little else. The steam from my tea swirls and glows under the desk lamp. Beyond the fence and the oak tree and the neighbor's slanted roof, the sky is just beginning to lighten.

Sitting at my desk, I see my patients: some of the men and women from my very first years in medical school, and the patients I cared for in residency, some of the sickest and dearest people I've ever known. Although in truth, I never really knew any of them, not as well as I should have.

One morning in my intern year, after working all night on Labor & Delivery, I saw a new patient, a thirty-four-year-old Filipina woman who spoke barely any English. I performed a vaginal ultrasound to date her pregnancy. It showed a miscarriage—a motionless fetus with no heartbeat—although she wasn't yet bleeding. She had walked into the clinic radiant, proud, expectant. "You see a baby?" she kept asking me. I said, "Just a second," and stepped out to get Dr. K. He strode into the room, took the probe from me and re-inserted it into the woman's vagina. His movements were more confident than mine, swift and blunt. I saw her wince.

He looked at the image and said to me, "Mm-hmm, I agree with you." The woman's eyes darted back and forth between us. Keeping the probe between her legs, Dr. K twirled the screen to show her. "You see this?" He pointed. "That's your baby. And unfortunately, there's no heartbeat. This pregnancy is not going to continue. So."

She turned to me, confused. "No baby?" Her mouth hung open.

My face burned. I wanted to yank Dr. K's tactless words from the air and grab the ultrasound probe from his hand. Instead I stood next to him, a silent accomplice. I also felt unfairly resentful of the woman. I'd thought all she would need from me was a shiny black-and-white picture, a congratulatory smile, a date on a calendar.

Now Dr. K was hurrying out of the room and leaving me alone with her, her broken English and her searching eyes. She sat up, pulling her legs into her chest to reveal the white dome of her bottom under the drape, flecked with coarse black hairs and smeared with ultrasound gel. I chose the kindest, simplest words I could think of: *There is a pregnancy, but it won't grow into a baby; you're going to bleed and it's going to come out.* She just sat there, hugging her knees, starting to cry. I tried to force myself to slow down, comfort her, concentrate. But I knew there was a line of patients in the waiting room and that I could not sleep until they had all been seen.

I really did try my best. I carved out the extra time where I could. But now I am beginning to think you need more than time to truly connect to another person. There is something else, a willingness and ability to reach across the space between you, to touch that person, not just physically, but touch them on the inside, and—this is the hard part—allow them to touch you, too.

After hibernating for the summer and fall, I have only just begun working again. In my first days as a full-fledged doctor, as I begin to care for patients—women and mothers—I can spend as much time with them as I need and want, here in the quiet dark of my little writing shed. Every evening after the harried pace of clinic, I have the luxury of returning to my husband and home, where time slows down. In the evenings, we cook and eat and drink. Sometimes after dinner Mo brings me a cup of tea, or I bring one to him. Other times we make love. In bed, our bodies find each other in a way they had forgotten—or at least mine had—over the previous three years.

In the predawn mornings I make my way to my shed, where I can visit again with the patients I cared for the day before, or a month ago, or three years ago. Here I can linger, talk with them, ask them questions I forgot or was too scared to ask when we sat face to face. The only thing I can't do is touch them. Sometimes I wish I could. But as I said, I am starting to think there must be other ways, besides the physical exam, to touch, and to be touched.

Before I'm due back in the clinic at the blessedly late hour of 8:30 a.m., I have only this to do. It is a slow process, but I think I am beginning to piece things together, one at a time.

I've made it here. After everything. I am a writer, a doctor, a wife. We have made a life together. It is the life I have dreamed of. It is almost complete.

PREVENTION

THE YEARS OF PREVENTION were long and ruthless—
but they were mine. They were years of purposeful
direction and control. I held my sights on the things
I most wanted, and my gaze was narrow. I was young.
But surely someone could have shown me the bigger
picture. All the well-meaning mentors in college
and medical school—many of them men, but some
women—who encouraged me to pursue my ambitions
as a writer and a doctor never once asked if I intended
to be a mother. They never told me to think about
when, if ever, the years of prevention would end.

Sometimes I think about what would have
happened if I'd quit.

Most people, at some point over the long years
of medical school and residency, flirt with the idea of

quitting. For me it wasn't just an occasional question mark on the daily routine of my training. It was a doubt that was with me always: when I rose before dawn; while I roamed the hospital hallways; when I pressed my stethoscope to a patient's back or watched the peculiar waveform of a jugular venous pulse in the beam of my flashlight; when I crawled into bed at night; and as I tossed for a fitful hour on a hospital couch, waiting for my pager to beep again.

I didn't mind working hard. But the work itself wasn't what I'd thought it would be. I knew about all the doctor-writers, and I clung to their names (William Somerset Maugham, William Carlos Williams, Anton Chekhov), even though not a single one of them was a woman. Through literature (Oliver Sacks, John Berger, Abraham Verghese), I had been seduced by a version of medicine that hardly exists anymore. I had wanted to use my knowledge and skills to guide patients from fear to safety, from suffering to relief. Instead I found myself working in the highly specialized, technological, and litigious world of hospital medicine in the United States, where the patient was the bothersome human being in a system centered around lab values, CT scans, and microbial cultures. As foolish as I felt admitting it, I had never liked science and math. I had been a creative writing major in college, and I was drawn to medicine for the humanity of it, the stories and the desire to see and touch people up close, to help them in their time of need. I resented spending hours poring through chemistry panels and antibiotic sensitivities.

But there was one month, and one patient in particular, that shined like a light for me through those dark years. It was the month I spent in my final year of medical school at the university's hospital-based abortion clinic. One Friday afternoon, just as the clinic was closing, a sixteen-year-old girl arrived at our door. She and her mother had driven from Nevada. "They said they can't help us there," her mother said. The girl's body bulged under her sweatshirt. She climbed onto an exam table and I slid the ultrasound probe over the curve of her abdomen to find the fetal heartbeat. "Hold that view steady," the attending doctor said to me, as he drew up the needle. The girl's eyes were on the ceiling, still and blue and brave, as the needle pierced her skin. Under my hands, that tiny heartbeat thrummed like a horse's gallop.

I suppose to most people it would have been a tragic case, one they would've liked to forget. But I clung to it. To me, what we did for that girl—the choice she made and the freedom we gave her to choose it— was exactly what I wanted to do as a doctor: to care for someone at a moment of her greatest vulnerability and fear, someone who didn't even expect to be treated with dignity, to help her across a precipice with my own hands.

There were plenty of times—most of the time, really—when I forgot about that patient and the care we gave her, when medical school was nothing but a slog. As graduation approached, I questioned whether I should continue on to internship and residency. But at that point, hundreds of thousands of dollars in debt and having spent five years of my life on this path, I didn't have the courage to make such a final decision.

So I opted for what was in many ways the easier choice, the path of least resistance: I continued.

In residency I was often awake at night and asleep in the middle of the day. Even when I wasn't working, I struggled to find a rhythm.

One cold and cloudy afternoon in early June at the end of my intern year, I awoke curled in an armchair in the living room to the sounds of neighborhood children playing in the street, a mother calling to them, a breeze stirring tree branches against a side window. Mo and I were living in a rented Spanish-style cottage in the city of Martinez, on the outskirts of the Bay Area. The house had a small lawn and two rose bushes out front that I hadn't pruned once since we'd moved in.

A week earlier Mo had told me, "I would like to feel more loved by you." This from the man whom I loved more than anything in the world. Our marriage was the one thing in my life that was exactly what I wanted, and I was on the verge of losing it.

I woke with a sadness that ached in my body like a virus. The clouds and the after-school time of day reminded me of napping on the couch as a little girl, waking from a deep, unexpected sleep to the shadows of evening, my parents' house with its familiar, muffled sounds and the knowledge that time had gone on without me, heedless of my sleep. Now, too, I had a feeling of being alone—not just alone in the house, which I didn't mind, but alone with this decision. I'd tried over and over again for years to make a choice: to stay or to quit? But I had done nothing but avoid and defer it, and now here I was.

That morning—it seemed like a lifetime ago, on the other side of my brief, deep afternoon sleep— after admitting patients all night to the hospital, I had knocked on the office door of our residency program director, Dr. Brennan. She waved me in. I told her about my conversation with my husband, and my concern that my marriage was at risk if I continued my residency. But I didn't stop there. I didn't pretend this was my only reason. I told her I'd been unhappy and unfulfilled, that

I doubted whether I was on the right path professionally. As a resident, I was under a contract to work, at minimum, until the end of the academic year the following July. Would it be possible, I asked, to leave sooner?

Dr. Brennan was shorter than I, with a no-nonsense blond bob and a small chin. Her blue eyes were as tired as those of any doctor—more tired, I thought, probably because her job was not just to care for patients, it was also to care for us, doctors in training. She knew our job wasn't easy. I knew her job wasn't easy either.

"Sit down," she said, pulling out two chairs and motioning me to join her. "I'm glad you came to me sooner rather than later."

Rubbing my eyes, I dragged myself out of the armchair, pulled on my tennis shoes and a hoodie and stepped out the front door into the fading daylight. Martinez is a small, mostly blue-collar city of oil refinery workers and longshoremen, with a heavy trade in methamphetamines. Our house was four short blocks from the county hospital and a half-mile from the waterfront, where a dirt path traced the edge of the bay. I set out in that direction, the wind in my face, walking quickly to reach my favorite spot before dark.

Near the end of the path, there was a place where the water curved close to the trail and the golden hills circled it like a bowl, where I could step across some rocks at low tide to one large, flat rock that jutted out into the water. I hopped out there and lowered myself down and let the waves lap the rocks under my feet. An orange container ship painted with huge Chinese characters passed in front of me, heading inland toward the port of Stockton. Behind me, geese in the marshy ponds honked and flapped their wings, settling in for the night.

I looked up at the hills where the sun threw its last slanted light, creating shadows like seams between folds in a blanket. The same thoughts, the same questions returned to me as they always did here, like the words of a familiar song from my childhood: *I know I will hear what I've heard before.* It occurred to me that my life as a resident was starting to feel familiar, with its own patterns and rituals. I could no longer count how many afternoons or early mornings I'd walked this path along the water, passing the hours until it was time to return to the hospital again. They all blurred together—like an afternoon nap on my parents' couch, or the feel of Mo's upper lip clinging to mine when we kissed, or the sound of crickets. I wondered whether even this moment was something I would one day feel nostalgic for, when it was only a memory.

Those evening sounds in my parents' house in Palo Alto: Mom in the kitchen, cooking and watching *The MacNeil/Lehrer NewsHour*; my sister on the phone upstairs; the dull, high-pitched buzz of Dad's table saw in the basement. They were the sounds of purposeful self-containment: four people tightly bound to one another but also, in a way, separate. "Everyone flies their own flag in your family," my friend Toby once said.

We ate dinner together every night at the dining table Dad built himself. There were four chairs, four plates of patterned Austrian china (no plastic for me and my sister, even when we were small children: "How else will you learn that if you drop a plate, it breaks?"), four cloth napkins rolled in their wooden rings. My ring bore a carved pattern of lines and squares. My sister Sabina's ring was wheat-colored with brown stripes. If a guest came over, a fifth napkin lay flat on the table next to a fifth plate. A fifth chair that didn't match the others was squeezed onto the end of the table.

Dad was big on table manners. He used to charge us a quarter every time he caught us leaning our bony elbows on the table. The salt and pepper shakers were passed together. There was always fresh bread in a woven basket, no butter. Dad poured the wine for himself and my mother. The milk was kept in a pitcher that matched the china. On pasta night, Sabina or I would grate the Parmesan cheese before dinner. It was passed around the table in a porcelain dish with a little spoon.

Napkins in our laps, child-size portions on our plates, my sister and I waited patiently until Dad raised his fork. Then we could take our first bite. Always hungry, I would sometimes stir the cheese into my pasta while I waited. If Dad noticed, he would scold me: "The fork has not been raised."

I put my hands in my lap, afraid of his anger.

Things were more relaxed before 5 p.m., when Dad was still at work. Every day he drove to the office in his boxy little BMW. He was a sinewy, salt-and-pepper-haired German engineer who ran a five-mile loop around the IBM business park every day at noon, showered in the janitorial office, and ate lunch alone at his desk: sardines on rye bread and a piece of fruit. On weekends, he ate the same lunch at home, plus a beer.

Mom worked from her home office while we played or did our homework. If one of us came home upset by some elementary school injustice, she stopped what she was doing and sat on the couch with us while we cried. "Oh honey," she would say, stroking my hair. "Oh baby. Oh pumpkin."

Mom's work in foreign aid took her to Asia and Africa several months out of the year. During that time, Dad tended to our needs. He took us to soccer practice and birthday parties and tucked us into bed with German lullabies. He sang to us tenderly, but the songs only made me miss Mom more, and I cried into my pillow after he left.

One afternoon when I was nine, I came home from school and went to the kitchen for my snack. My mom was home. Through the windows of the kitchen door, I saw my dad sitting on the back porch, head in his hands, staring down at the boards he had nailed in place that summer.

I went to my mom's office. "Why is Daddy home from work early?" I asked.

"Your *Lieber Opa* died today," my mom answered. "Daddy's very sad."

"Oh."

I ate my snack, finished my homework, watched a 30-minute TV show with my sister. It grew dark outside and my mom asked me to set the table. The windowpanes in the kitchen were fogged with boiling pasta water. I peered out and saw my dad still sitting there, that blank, troubled look on his face. But I didn't see him shed a single tear.

A few weeks later, I picked up the phone and heard my mom already on the line. She was talking to my aunt Margaret, her youngest sister, who had just returned from a prenatal ultrasound in which she had learned that there was "something wrong" with her unborn daughter. (Later she told me the diagnosis was Trisomy 18.) Margaret was sobbing into the phone, explaining that the only choices the doctors had given her were to abort the baby, or give birth to a very sick child who would die within days.

I listened for half an hour to her gasping sobs, my hand pressed over the mouthpiece. My mom's voice remained calm, comforting. If she felt any empathic horror at the thought of the doomed child living in her sister's belly, she never betrayed it. "Oh honey," she said, her voice soothing and steady. "Oh sweetie, oh honey."

My periods began late—at sixteen. For the rest of high school and college I bled sporadically, if at all. Instead of time being marked by a monthly period, it was marked by semesters, midterm exams, and standardized tests.

I was told this was common for women on my mother's side of the family. According to my aunt Margaret, our grandmother even had a "rather anti-feminist" theory about it: When a woman was working hard on intellectual pursuits, her body would "get the signal" and stop ovulating—the implication being that she couldn't possibly create a baby and pursue her education or career ambitions at the same time.

So for many years, "prevention" did not necessarily mean "birth control." I did eventually start birth control pills in college. Later, in the short interval between my wedding and the start of residency, I went to the university student health office and requested a Mirena IUD, which I had learned, in medical school, was a highly reliable form of long-acting contraception. The nurse practitioner inserted the IUD through my vagina and cervix with a tiny plastic applicator, a procedure I would eventually learn and perform thousands of times for other women. The little hormone-infused rod sat in my uterus for the next three years, where it zapped my libido and dried up my periods as well as my vaginal fluids. During residency, even on the rare nights when I was at home and awake, sex with Mo felt like I was being split open and scraped with sandpaper. I would cry out and roll away, exhausted and ashamed.

In my junior year of college I took leave for a semester to go to India, alone. I had found a volunteer position teaching English in a rural village school.

A day or two before I was to fly, I was packing my backpack in the late afternoon. My dad approached me holding a small white box. Inside the box was a pill. He wanted me to take this pill to India in case I somehow got pregnant while I was there. He may have used the word "rape" or implied it. I can't recall his exact words, but knowing my dad, I'm sure he made himself clear. He told me he had requested this pill from my cousin, a doctor in Germany, and I vaguely understood that it must have been "RU-486," the abortion pill that had been legal in Europe for some time, but, in 2003, had been only recently approved by the U.S. Food and Drug Administration. Probably my dad didn't know exactly how the pill worked or how it should be taken; in any case, he didn't give me specific instructions.

"Dad." I gave him my best *how-could-you-be-so-stupid* face. "I don't even get my period." But I could tell he didn't follow my reasoning: that even if I were to have sex in India, even if I were raped, I wouldn't get pregnant.

Instead he heard me saying, *Daddy, I'm your little girl. I've never ever had sex and I never will.*

"Well," he said, holding my stare, "I want you to take it with you anyway."

Other than being the cause for this embarrassing exchange, that pill meant nothing to me. At the very least it was a nuisance, an extra ounce of weight to carry in my backpack around the subcontinent. At most, it was a symbol of that fierce self-reliance that our parents had come to expect from us: If I found myself pregnant, alone, in India, I would have everything I needed to deal with it myself.

Eventually I flushed the pill down a toilet in New Delhi, shortly before flying home. Another careless first-world disposal of something that to another woman, in another life, would have been worth more than gold.

When my college friend Angie was in Bali a few years later on a prestigious teaching fellowship, she got pregnant by her Balinese boyfriend. Abortion is illegal in Indonesia. Angie later told me about the terror and urgency of the following days, waiting and searching, not knowing whom she could trust or what would be done to her body.

The boyfriend took her to a neighborhood doctor who told her, "You shouldn't be doing this, but take these pills and you won't be pregnant anymore." She took the pills. She waited. Nothing happened. She called her parents, who said they'd fly there as soon as they could.

She went to a different clinic, where she'd heard a lot of American expats received medical care. She was led into a quiet, "sterile-looking" room and put to sleep. When she woke up, she wasn't pregnant anymore.

By the time her parents arrived, Angie's abortion was already over. But at least they got on a plane. At least they stayed by her side afterward, while she bled and cried and stared at the white walls of their hotel room.

My dad gave me a pill in a cardboard box.

The summer after I graduated from college, our family spent two weeks in Germany for what would be our last vacation together. We convened from the four corners of the globe: Sabina was living and working in China at the time; my mom was in North Africa on business; I was working on a farm in Tuscany. Only my dad flew in from our home in California. We visited family and vacationed in the Bavarian countryside, hiking and swimming in a lake under the silver mountains. At the end of the trip, we went our separate ways: Sabina flew back to China, my mom and

I returned to California, and my dad stayed behind for a few days to visit with his sisters and friends. During that short window—a warm, sunny weekend in August in Berlin—my dad suffered a stroke.

None of us flew back to Germany to be with him. Mom said it wasn't necessary; his sisters were there to look after him. Dad agreed. He stayed in the hospital, the left side of his body weak and limp, until the doctors declared him safe to fly. My mom and I met him at the San Francisco airport, where a flight attendant wheeled him off the plane.

When I was nine, watching my dad in the blue light of the early evening, waiting for him to shed a tear for his father, I turned to my mom and asked her if she believed in heaven.

She was standing at the silverware drawer, pulling out four knives, four forks, a little spoon. I had the feeling she already knew her answer, that she had thought about what she believed and about what she would tell me when I asked. She handed me the little bundle of silverware, the warm imprint of her hands lingering on the stainless steel.

"I don't believe heaven is a place," she said. "I think that in life, we're limited by our bodies. We can't see each other or trust each other completely.

So in heaven, the boundaries of our bodies sort of ...
disappear. We're no longer trapped. Our souls float free,
and we can connect with each other and love each
other perfectly."

I am still comforted by the idea of heaven as a state,
a set of conditions. But if our family is, as my friend
Toby said, defined by its boundaries—both around us,
our little nucleus, and between us—then my mom's
heaven is, in a way, a place without family. It is a place
to break all the rules we've lived by, rules we've set
for ourselves and those set for us by others. In a place
where babies don't die, nor are they born, there are
no mothers and there are no children. Discipline and
self-reliance mean nothing; generosity means nothing.
Nobody hurts or touches anyone else, because there is
nothing to touch—except one soul to another, perfect
and deep.

A story can begin almost anywhere. Here I am trying to write about my medical training and instead I'm writing about my parents' house and my childhood: my dad's strict rules at the dinner table, my aunt Margaret's abortion, and my mom's idea of heaven.

But there is another beginning, too.

I was having sex in college, no matter what my dad thought or what I might have let him believe.

Mo and I met on the first day of my freshman year. He was a sophomore, the RA assigned to my hall. Later he used to say about his first year, before I arrived, "That was before you were born." I loved when he said that; it made me feel as though his life began when he met me. But of course, it means just the opposite: My life began when I met him.

By summer vacation, we were a couple.

I don't think I know the difference between knowing Mo and being in love with him. I was just a child when we met—seventeen years old. That's not the kind of difference you can know or remember.

Mo is the only son of two doctors, immigrants from the Indian state of Punjab. He was pre-med from his first day of college ("before I was born"). Late at night, after I and the rest of the admiring freshmen dispersed from his room, he would pull out his biology textbook and his stacks of organic chemistry equations. Walking to the bathroom with my toothbrush, I saw him hunched over his desk, his square jaw and thick brow lit by the glow of his desk lamp.

On breaks from school, we spent as much time together as we could, visiting each other in the homes where we grew up. Mo fit in easily with my family, as he did everywhere, adapting to our quiet rhythms. In the afternoons, he sat with his laptop while my mom and I read on the couch. When my dad brought him a beer—room temperature, the way Dad liked them—he drank it happily. At the dinner table he listened to the conversation, asking questions, adding a few remarks when prompted. Afterwards he helped carry dishes to the kitchen; he asked my mom how she liked the plates loaded in the dishwasher. Then he joined us for our favorite family movies on the tiny television set: *Home Alone*, *Fawlty Towers*, anything starring Julie Andrews.

In Mo's parents' house, there was no dinner table. There was an enormous kitchen counter, wide and long as a cruise ship, with plates piled like smokestacks in the center. Platters of food were continuously reheated to feed anyone at any time. A canister of hot chai was refilled throughout the day by one of Mo's grandmothers, who shuffled around the kitchen in their saris.

Mo's parents were the first in their families to leave India. When they were barely settled in Sacramento, they sponsored their own parents and siblings, one household at a time, to join them in the U.S. As Mo and his two sisters describe their childhood, there was always some combination of cousins, aunts, uncles, and grandparents living in their home, often for months at a time, until they gradually settled and moved into nearby homes of their own. In Mo's family, everyone was welcome. There was no schedule; there were no boundaries. There was no beginning and no end. There were no guests. Even I, Mohit's "friend" from college, was treated like family. Nothing could have been more different from the house where I grew up.

In addition to all the aunts and uncles and cousins, a crowd that to me always felt like a small party, there were the real parties. The house was a Daddy Warbucks–style mansion, originally built as the governor's residence, and designed for entertaining.

CHRISTINE HENNEBERG

Mo's parents threw huge parties, packing the house with people. Hired waiters served catered Indian food and unlimited alcohol. Before the guests arrived, Mo's mom would wrap me in a gold-edged sari and adorn me with diamonds. Mo protested, "She's not Bollywood Barbie, Mom." But later he slipped his hands under the silk pleats at my waist and told me I looked beautiful.

There is a certain type of boundless generosity that you don't often see in this country, maybe in this world. An openness and inclusivity that makes you feel at home even where you are a stranger, where nobody owes you anything.

Mo's room was at the end of the hall, with its own attached bathroom. His mom always laid out two sets of towels before we arrived. The room held a large-screen TV, a king-sized bed where we made love like movie stars, and a walk-in closet. Inside the closet was the family *mandir,* or temple. Brightly colored posters and statues of Hindu deities were strung with flashing Christmas lights and garlands of marigolds. Scattered among these were photographs of dead relatives; drawings of heavy-lidded Sikh gurus in orange turbans; a jade Buddha sitting in the center of a Lotus flower; the Virgin Mary, her eyes downcast; and a wooden carving of Christ on the cross.

In Mo's bed at night, I felt those gods watching over us as we slept, and I wanted to lie with him forever under their benevolent, fluorescent glow.

In addition to all the extended family who came and went, Mo and his sisters grew up with two cousins, Aanand and Neil, who spent much of their childhoods in Mo's parents' house. Mo called them his "cousin-brothers." Aanand was Mo's age, Neil about five years younger. Their father had suffered a ruptured aneurysm when Aanand and Neil were very young; it left him barely able to walk or talk. Their mother soon took him back to India, where she could afford full-time care. Neil initially went to India with his parents, but he returned to the U.S. for high school. Mo's parents raised Aanand and Neil in their home, like their own sons—although the two boys attended public schools and, later, state universities, while Mo and his sisters were sent to private schools and elite liberal arts colleges.

I do not mean that Aanand and Neil weren't loved—they were. Only that these were the facts that were visible to me. I made meaning of them however I could, like a person on another planet watching the shadows on the face of the moon.

The first time I met Neil was during a winter vacation in college. After greeting Mo's parents and sisters and several other family members, Mo and I carried our bags to Mo's bedroom. Down the hallway in a small den, a TV screen flickered in the dark. Mo ducked his head in. "Hey, Neil," he said, his voice friendly but self-conscious. Neil lifted his chin off his chest to look at us. His eyes were hooded and dark. His shoulders sloped into his thick torso like a large sea animal. He clutched a remote control with both hands, his forearms between his knees.

"How are you, man?" Mo said. Neil rose from the couch and immediately bent to touch Mo's feet with his fingertips. "Oh my gosh, Neil, stop it," Mo said, laughing, grabbing Neil's right hand in his and pumping it, pulling him upright. "Good to see you. How've you been?" Then without pausing, "This is Chrissy."

Neil did not look at me, or touch my feet. His eyebrows were so thick, I would have had to crouch down to see the whites of his eyes. He mumbled something to Mo in Hindi, then looked back at the remote control on the couch.

"Alright, we'll see you later, man," Mo said, and waved me on down the hall.

Just like that, I became complicit in Mo's approach to Neil, which perhaps was the approach of his whole family—or at least that was how I saw it at the time. I was acutely aware of the loneliness that wafted from that dark room, like the smell of something rotten. But I pretended to ignore it.

Mo and I remained a couple after college, but our medical training kept us three thousand miles apart. He completed medical school and residency in Washington, D.C., where he lived in a split-level home in Georgetown. I attended the Joint Medical Program at UC Berkeley and UCSF. I lived in a small studio apartment in North Oakland, near the Ashby BART station and the Berkeley Bowl. In some ways, this arrangement was easier than living together. It allowed us both to focus our attention entirely on our medical studies, except for one or two weekends a month when we would fly across the country to see each other.

I never loved medical school. I got good grades, but the science didn't interest me. During the first few years, I woke every morning at 5:30 to write for an hour before biking to class at 8 a.m. From my bed, I could reach my diary on my nightstand and the cord for the blinds, which zipped up to reveal an east-facing window and, outside, a dense birch tree whose leaves filtered the morning sunlight. In the evening, I sat at my desk and studied, waiting for Mo to call me on Skype when he returned from the hospital. I missed him, but I had a comfortable enough routine of writing, attending class, and studying.

When I began working in the hospital, things got more interesting, because there were patients to talk to and actual bodies to examine. Nevertheless, some of my most vivid memories are not of patients, but of my own fears and mistakes.

On my first day as a student on the hospital's internal medicine service, the intern gave me a brief rundown of the weekly schedule: which days we were on call, when the important conferences and Grand Rounds took place, and resident-led educational activities. "This Thursday, if we're finished by 6 p.m., there's Journal Club in the cafeteria conference room," he said. "Med students are welcome to join. It's usually pretty good."

"Great!" I said. "I'll be there!" That Thursday morning I packed my diary in my hospital bag. I hurried to complete my work and made my way to the conference room, eager to write. Inside, a group of residents were already gathered, eating off cafeteria trays and looking tired in their rumpled white coats. One resident was standing at the head of the table with a stack of photocopies. He handed one to me. "Hopefully you've read it already," he said. I looked down at the article. It bore the red-and-gold banner of *The New England Journal of Medicine* and was titled something like, "Chronic Thromboembolic Pulmonary Hypertension."

"Thanks," I mumbled, and slouched into a chair, realizing my mistake. *Journal Club.* They weren't here to write down their deepest thoughts and feelings. They were here to discuss an article in a medical journal. But I was too self-conscious to leave. For two hours, the residents debated the merits and flaws of the article and the study it described, critiquing its statistical methods and its conclusions.

It was nearly 9 p.m. by the time I got home. I had missed a Skype call from Mo.

I signed online.

"Where were you?" he asked. "Hard day?"

I explained my mistake, cursing myself for not being brave enough to leave the meeting. It was too late now to write before bed—I had to be at the hospital by six the next morning.

Instead of laughing, he comforted me. "Oh Chrissy. I'm sorry. You must have been miserable, sitting there listening to them talk about pulmonary hypertension."

I pressed my eyelids together, shaking my head. "It's just ... I can feel it slipping away, you know? I sit down to write ... and nothing comes out. It's like I'm losing my words."

He shook his head, reached out to touch the camera on his computer as though he were touching my face. The whorls of his fingerprints pressed against my screen. "Don't worry about that now," he said. "Your words aren't going anywhere."

One spring weekend when Mo was out visiting, his parents came over for lunch at my apartment. As I remember it, Mo's "cousin-brother" Neil came along with them. He sat quietly in a chair in the living room, enormous, unblinking, like a circus lion perched on a stool, at once pitiful and dignified.

After lunch, Mo's mom made chai. His dad pulled up his calendar on his phone. They told us they needed to set a date at least a year in advance for the size and scale of the wedding they were planning for us. They would need to clean the house from top to bottom, prepare the garden, polish the chandeliers. They would have to book the horse trainer and the *mhendi* artist who would tattoo my hands and feet. "She is very popular," Mo's mother said, wagging her head. "Families are booking her *two* years in advance."

Mo and I weren't even engaged at that point, although we'd talked about it. We shrugged and agreed to Memorial Day weekend of the following year. Mo proposed to me a few weeks later, and we laughed and rolled our eyes at the thought of his parents already planning seating arrangements. But I also felt something had been taken from us, a sense of privacy and ownership over the life we were making together.

"Maybe," I said to Mo one night on Skype, when I was lying alone in my bed, "we could have a small wedding. Something intimate, just our families, a few of our close friends."

Mo actually laughed. "I don't think that's gonna fly, Chrissy."

"Why not? Your parents have plenty of chances to throw big parties. They do it all the time. And there will be other weddings: Your sisters …"

"Yeah, but … I know my parents. This is what they want."

"But what about what we want?"

He sighed. "Chrissy. I care about what you want. But my parents … They've always done everything for me, you know? They've given me everything. This is the chance to let them …"

"Let them what?" I said. *Let them show off?*

"It's a chance to let them know how much we appreciate them, everything they've done for us."

I looked down at my feet and hands stretched out in front of me. I tried to imagine them decorated in bridal henna, the intricate brown patterns that would wrap around my wrists and ankles, reaching all the way up the curve of my calves, the nooks and crannies of my elbows. I thought of my parents. They had never been to a single one of Mo's parents' parties, although Mo's parents always pressed them with invitations. I imagined them at our enormous wedding, lost in a sea of bodies—turbaned men drunk with whiskey, bangled and bejeweled women wrapped in saris. My mom would be pale and fragile, my dad tottering on his cane, straining to read lips, trying not to show his confusion.

"Hey," Mo said, tapping the camera. "You okay?"

"Yeah." I smiled at the image of him on the screen.

In the months leading up to the wedding, Neil began "acting strange," as Mo said.

"*More* strange?" I said, aware that I was walking a thin line between honest and intrusive. Mo said nothing, and I dropped it. We rarely talked about Neil, even though we saw him often. He was finishing up college that year, and it seemed to me he spent a lot of time with Mo's parents—perhaps because he was friendless, perhaps because they were worried about him. Whenever we visited them in Sacramento, Neil was wandering around the house as he always had, his head down, mumbling in Hindi, speaking only when spoken to.

Mo had told me about little incidents that had occurred while Neil was in high school and college: strange obsessions he'd had with his weight, dieting, Catholicism. At least once, some jewelry went missing from the house. Mo tracked it down easily on eBay, where Neil had posted it for auction. When Mo's dad asked him about it, Neil didn't seem defensive or ashamed. He said he'd planned to send the money to his parents in India.

One day that spring, Mo was out in California. We were planning to spend the weekend in Sacramento, meeting with his parents and the wedding planner. In the car on the way there, Mo told me Neil had been hospitalized recently on a brief psychiatric hold. He didn't know the details, except that Neil had been visiting his brother Aanand in L.A. the weekend before. After Neil spent a couple days "acting strange," Aanand was concerned enough to take him to the closest emergency room. During a psych evaluation, it came out that Neil had bought a gun.

"He has a *gun*?" I said, making my eyes big for emphasis.

"That's what my dad said."

"Where is he now?"

"At my parents' house."

"And where is the gun?"

Mo let out a breath. "He was keeping it at my parents' house. But they made him get rid of it. I think they sold it or something."

"Oh, great. So then … what? He's all better now?"

"I think so. Yeah."

"You think so."

We didn't stay at Mo's parents' house that night. In the late evening, after the wedding planner had left, I sat with Mo and held his hand in mine. "It's not that I don't feel safe here," I said.

He said, "What do you want to do?"

We packed our things and drove twenty minutes to the nearest Marriott Courtyard. Mo called his dad from the car.

"What did he say?" I asked.

"He didn't make a big deal out of it at all. He just said, 'I understand and I don't blame you.' He told me to use his points to pay for the room."

In the bed with its cold, crisp sheets, I lay next to Mo and watched the flicker of the TV screen on his eyes. He didn't lace his fingers with mine when I took his hand under the covers. I didn't know if he was angry with me or worried about Neil or depressed by the Merlot-colored curtains, the sound of forced air from the heating vent. Maybe he was just homesick at that hotel on the outskirts of Sacramento, close to his family but not with them. I lay there listening to the hum and rattle of the air behind the walls, and I realized I was homesick, too.

The following weekend I drove to Palo Alto to see my parents. My mom and I took a walk in the early morning. The daffodils were in bloom and the tips of the tree branches were studded with pale green. "What do you think I should have done?" I asked her.

"I think you did the right thing. Absolutely the right thing." Her eyes were fixed straight ahead of her, arms swinging emphatically at her sides. She wore sweats and a UCSF sweatshirt; her short, silver-blond hair bounced with each step. "I'm glad you had the presence of mind, you know, to do what you did. If you had told me before you went up there, I would've said the same thing. I would have forbid you to stay there."

"Mom. Forbid me?"

"Well, I mean it. Who knows what could happen? I mean, not just now. What about the wedding?"

The wedding was two months away, and it was the first time my mom had brought it up unprompted. She and my dad were only marginally involved in the plans. Usually she just listened while I complained about the ever-expanding guest list, four-hour meetings with the wedding planner, the cost of the bridal saris and the jewelry Mo's mom wanted me to wear. His parents were paying for everything.

"What about the wedding?" I said.

"Well, is Neil going to be at the wedding?"

"Of course he's going to be there."

"And is he going to bring a gun? Is he going to have another psychiatric breakdown at the wedding?"

"Mom. No. The gun is gone."

"The gun is gone. Fine. But he knows where to get a gun if he wants one. Is he in therapy? Is he taking medication?"

I had never heard my mom use the word "therapy."

I sighed. My breath made a cloud in the clear, cold air. "I don't think so," I said. "Neil has, you know, refused therapy before, and I think he's refusing now. Refusing to take meds, too."

"But this is different than before. He didn't have a gun before."

I shrugged.

"What? Did he?"

"No. I don't know. I don't know! I don't think anyone knows anymore."

"Well, now they know something. They have to do something now."

"I guess they can't force him."

"Can't force him?" There was a wavering edge of something—fear, helplessness—in her voice. "They're his parents. Or if they're not his real parents, at least they're responsible for him. They could set some rules, some consequences. I don't understand that family sometimes. They can't force Neil to take psych meds, but they can force you and Mo to have a four-day wedding that you don't even want? Who is in charge in this family? Who owes what to whom?"

I stayed quiet for some time, thinking. We had crossed at the traffic light a few blocks from home and descended into the woody acres of the Stanford campus. Eucalyptus branches arched over our heads like fans waved by royal attendants, their scent wafting down on us. A reedy graduate student in jogging shorts approached us, drawing closer, then receding in the distance like a ship on the ocean. It was all as familiar as the rhythm of my mom's breath between her words and her footsteps.

I had an urge to take her hand, to stand still and face her, even cry—but we kept walking. She was entirely missing the point, I thought, yet in her practical and misguided way, I sensed she was trying to protect me, to shelter me from some still unmeasured danger.

I remember our wedding as being full of joy and sadness and, perhaps, secret relief. Neil was not there. We were told not to mention his name; if anyone asked, we said, "He couldn't be here." But honestly, I don't remember anyone asking about Neil.

I had never seen Mo's parents' house so packed with people. They were, as always, the perfect host and hostess, generous and gregarious. My parents and sister were the picture of composure: my father in his wheelchair, Sabina attending to him, my mother discreet and smiling.

Mo and I circled the sacred fire, each bare-footed step a symbol of the journeys we would take together. Afterward we danced under a pale evening sky, on the slope of the hill that swept down to the American River below us, the water sparkling in the dusk. We clung to each other in our happiness, our relief, our desperation. I don't know what we felt, really, because we never spoke of it—not that day, and not afterwards.

Two weeks later, finished with his medical training, Mo left Washington D.C. We moved into our little cottage in Martinez, and I began my residency.

TRYING

IT IS SPRING NOW, the mornings still cold but the sun rising earlier. Every day I tell myself, *You are happy with your life just as it is. Enjoy this time. There's no reason to be impatient.*

I am enjoying it. I don't want anything to change. But it's hard to be patient.

When we returned from Barcelona in early September, I called up my friends whose texts and voicemails I had left unanswered during the three years of residency. They'd all promised me they understood, that they would still be there when my training was finished. Home now, free, I thought we would resume the friendships I remembered: eat a lazy Sunday brunch together, plan a girls' weekend in Palm Springs, go out dancing.

My best friend Jana and I met for a walk. Jana's mom had died that January, following a sudden diagnosis of gastric cancer. She was 68. I'd managed to get a morning off to attend the funeral. I sat behind Jana, who looked tiny and sheltered between her dad and sister, the ridges of her shoulder blades tenting her dark blouse.

On our walk, Jana looked happier than I'd seen her in a long time. We followed a trail along the bay that reminded me of the trail in Martinez. She asked me about my plans for work after residency. I was full of ideas of what I wanted my career and my life to look like: writing, abortion work, women's health, teaching. She supplied generous enthusiasm for all of it, encouraging me to schedule and protect time for my writing.

I should have known she was bursting with her own excitement, her own visions. I suppose in a way I did know. When we reached the end of the trail and turned back, the wind whipping our hair in our faces, I asked, "So what's new with you?"

"Well," she said, "I'm pregnant."

I exclaimed and hugged her, pried her with all the necessary, excited questions. I could not tell her then, any more than I could have told her on the day of her mom's funeral, the perverse jealousy I felt: a selfish, paradoxical desire to catch up to something I had long regarded with dreadful resignation. *If it has to happen, at least don't leave me behind while you go on without me.*

Jana's mom—whose high heels had tapped down the hallway while I lay awake in my sleeping bag on the floor of Jana's room, who had cooked David Eyre's pancakes for us Sunday mornings, sprinkling powdered sugar through a sifter like snow—was dead. She had been sick for exactly one year, and now she was gone. Jana and her dad and sister seemed to have grown closer through all of it, gathering around each other like birds in a storm. Meanwhile our family drifted on in the purgatory of Dad's slow, bitter decline. There was no unity in it, only division, resentment, and exhaustion.

And now Jana was pregnant. It seemed to me that by going first, she would necessarily have the easier time of it. I imagined that after she passed through the gates of motherhood they would begin to slowly draw shut behind her, leaving only a narrow gap through which I might slip into safety.

It turned out they were all pregnant: Jana, Margot, and Susannah (who had had one miscarriage that summer and was pregnant again). Angie, the friend whose first pregnancy had ended with an illegal abortion in Bali, had had her first baby while Mo and I were in Spain: a girl, born by C-section at the same hospital where I'd trained as a medical student. The only one not yet pregnant was Toby. She and her wife had undergone thirteen rounds of intrauterine insemination with donor sperm. A fertility specialist had recently suggested moving on to IVF, which would be more invasive but had higher rates of successful pregnancy. "So this could be it," Toby told me hopefully over the phone. "Once we have the embryos, we'll be more than halfway there."

What else was there to do? Shortly before Christmas I removed my IUD. (Confident and impatient, I reached up my vagina and tried to yank it out with my own forefinger and thumb. Nothing budged. So I went to Planned Parenthood, where a nurse practitioner took it out with one quick tug.)

It seems there won't ever be a "better" time, and there might be no other time at all, since I'm now thirty-three years old. I've gone from ambivalence and dread to suddenly, desperately wanting something—if not a baby, then at least to know that the possibility is available to me. But I'm beginning to think perhaps those gates have already slammed shut, leaving me behind.

It's been three months since the IUD came out. And for the third time, I'm bleeding.

We were taught in medical school that when a pregnant woman presents for her first prenatal visit, before congratulating her you should ask, "Is this a planned pregnancy?" Make room for a conversation about her options, in case this is not a pregnancy she wants to continue.

Yesterday I saw a young woman, twenty-five years old and pregnant for the first time. "Is this a planned pregnancy?" I asked.

She looked confused, almost suspicious. "Well, uh, no? I mean I wasn't using birth control. But I wasn't exactly planning it either."

"Well, are you happy about it?" I asked her.

"Yeah," she said. "I am."

We were looking at each other across a gulf of difference and misunderstanding. I could not imagine being happy about something I had not purposefully chosen. She was perhaps thinking, *What is this doctor talking about? How do you* plan *a pregnancy? Does she have some kind of control over her body that I don't?*

I, too, am beginning to wonder what I mean by that question. Usually I am so careful with my language. But this is something ambiguous and misleading. To *want* and to *plan* are not the same thing.

The problem with the question we were taught in medical school is this: The opposite of prevention is not planning. "Birth control" is a wonderful thing, and it does give you some type of control. But what about when birth is what you want? Then where is the control? I cannot plan a pregnancy any more than I can plan which angels and demons appear in my dreams. I know as well as anyone that there are no guarantees.

So far, every single heterosexual friend of mine who has tried has been able to conceive. Statistically speaking, *someone* has to be the one who can't get pregnant. Wouldn't it just be the most horrible and ironic thing in the world if it turns out to be me—the abortion doctor?

I made a dinner reservation last week, before my period began, when I thought Mo and I might celebrate a belated Valentine's Day and perhaps a positive pregnancy test. But it's raining and I'm bleeding, and Valentine's Day, as usual, seems like a cruel joke.

At the restaurant, over expensive cocktails, I tell Mo my big secret: my IUD is out. We are trying. We have been trying, actually, for three months.

But it turns out it isn't a secret at all. As usual, he is on to me.

"Yeah, I kind of suspected that," he says.

"Why?"

He mentions that I've seemed especially "motivat-ed" to have sex lately. I even got mad at him one night when he promised he was coming to bed but didn't. I remember that night: the ovulation predictor kit had flashed "HIGH" that morning. Oh! I was so pissed at him for that whole long hour, lying there in the dark, waiting. Eventually I came stomping out in my slippers to find him still on the couch, reading the news on his laptop.

I tell him I'm starting to worry. I thought he would stroke my hair and say, *Don't worry, Chrissy, you'll get pregnant and everything's going to be fine.*

Instead he admits he's a little worried, too. I didn't expect him to say that, and I tell him so.

"You know me," he says. "I worry about everything." And it's true.

But this is exactly what I don't want: for both of us to be worried.

What he's worried about, he says, is that if we can't have kids, it might turn out to be his "fault," and that I will resent him for it. I promise him it won't be like that. "If we can't have kids," I say, "the reason doesn't matter. We're in this together, so whether it's your body or my body doesn't make a difference. This is our family."

But of course, I am terrified of the same thing: that it could be my "fault."

"It's not just about being a woman," I tell him. "I think all women feel this way—like it would be some kind of curse or dirty secret. And I know that's not true. It's just … I don't know if I would be able to keep doing my work. I would worry so much about what people would think. About the reason."

"What do you mean? What reason?"

"You know, the work I do, and the idea that … You know how your mom is so superstitious? I'm afraid if we keep trying and trying, after a while she'll figure it out, you know? That we're having a hard time. And she'll suggest that maybe if I stop doing abortions …" When I say that, suddenly the tears come and I can't stop. It's embarrassing, sitting there in the restaurant, crying like a child. For the first time I realize how scared I've been. Not just about the idea of infertility, but about the reason.

The abortion doctor who can't get pregnant. It would make a good premise for a novel.

But where does that fear come from? What does it mean about my true feelings about the work I do, that I would even entertain the idea of some kind of karmic punishment—for what? For not taking seriously enough the value of a "life"?

Every woman is different, and every moment in each of our lives is different. If I had gotten pregnant in the middle of medical school, it would have felt like a disaster. I probably would have gotten an abortion.

But of course that never happened—because I was so careful, so smart. Or so I thought.

And now that the years of prevention are over, I suddenly see my patients in a new light. They have something I want. And I doubt myself.

Only a month into my intern year (the first year of residency), I felt like an occupying soldier in a conflict zone. We were the privates, the conscripts. They'd thrown us in with minimal training, supposedly to use our skills and tools in matters of life and death. But we spent most of our time performing mundane daily tasks in order to survive and support the mission, tasks we hadn't been trained to do and barely understood.

Every morning: an alarm at 4:45 a.m. A short shower and a five-minute walk to the hospital, where the red EMERGENCY sign glowed like a flare at the top of the hill. In an overheated room full of computers, I reviewed morning lab results while gnawing on a banana and the paper rim of a coffee cup, its pulp on my tongue.

Morning rounds, 6:30 a.m.: A ninety-year-old woman with a broken hip, delirious from her medications, her pain, and the unfamiliar surroundings of the surgical unit. Bright lights, beeping IV poles, nurses laughing and joking in a dozen different accents. Frightened and alone, she cried out as I lifted the corner of her sheet to prod at her hip. I barely knew what to look for under her bandage. A 46-year-old man with uncontrolled diabetes had had his leg amputated below the knee to halt a spreading bone infection. He had an autistic daughter at home; he asked me to help find a caretaker for her until he could walk again. Two nurses offered me a bite of Filipino sweet bread while I waited at their desk for a fax from another hospital, the records of an elderly woman with a fresh surgical scar on her abdomen and no memory of how it got there. A particular stretch of hallway reeked with the yellow, medicated smell of diarrhea. The P.A. system beeped three times for a Code Blue. If I was lucky, it was someone else's patient dying. If I was unlucky, I'd spend the morning transferring a pale, clammy body to the ICU, a tube stuck down its throat, or filling out death paperwork and calling the next of kin: *Something unexpected … Please come in as soon as you possibly can …*

8 a.m. lecture: Over a hospital cafeteria breakfast, an attending physician, just a year out of residency himself, lectured our group of twelve residents on the functions and dysfunctions of the renal nephron, his voice punctuated every few minutes by the mechanical beep of a pager. Bleary-eyed, we rose one at a time to dial the number flashing on our screens: A radiology tech needed someone to replace the order for an

abdominal CT scan—it should have been ordered with contrast. The lab reported a "critical" hemoglobin value of 4.2 for a leukemia patient on hospice who shouldn't have had his blood drawn in the first place. A social worker explained regretfully that a homeless man with multiple myeloma would be in the hospital one more day—she couldn't find a nursing home to take him.

Most afternoons, I hustled across the parking lot to see patients in my primary care clinic, or if I was on call I continued working in the hospital, tying up loose ends, answering pages, admitting new patients from the emergency room. By 6 p.m. I hoped to be on my way home, but most days it was closer to nine, sometimes later. Then back up in the morning before sunrise.

These were the days on the general inpatient unit, where interns spent about eight months of the year. The rest of the year was split between two months on the "outpatient" service, seeing patients in clinic only, and two months on Labor & Delivery, where we delivered babies all day, all night, sometimes both.

The hospital often felt like a war zone, but I quickly decided I was no soldier. I was something else: an embedded reporter, there to learn and to perform the basic functions as part of the team. I was there, in a way, to serve—but not in the role they thought I was serving. I was not one of them, and I didn't want to be initiated or to belong. I was there to witness and to write it down. When this was all over and they sent us home, I would have something to take with me. I would have the stories.

It was easy to get lost in the hospital. Within a few months I knew the hallways like the neighborhood streets I'd biked as a child, where I navigated by the color of the houses and the shapes of the fence posts. Still I could lose track of exactly where I was—what unit, what floor, what time it was, what day it was—especially in the middle of the night.

I was vaguely aware that I was on the fifth floor when I was called to pronounce the patient dead. It was clear from when I arrived early that evening that she was getting close: a seventy-three-year-old woman with advanced dementia and aggressive bladder cancer. I called her daughter, Theresa, at the start of my shift, to let her know she may want to spend the night here with her mother. She seemed to have taken a turn toward what we called "actively dying."

It was an unusual place for a patient to die: 5-D, the low-acuity "med-surg" unit on the fifth floor. These rooms were mostly filled with patients needing or recovering from acute procedures—cholecystectomies, appendectomies. The kind of patients an intern could look after.

I was just finishing a post-operative exam on a young man who had had a routine gallbladder surgery, when the nurse approached me. "Doctor, the patient in Bed 32."

I didn't look up. Bed numbers meant nothing to me. "Mm-hmm? What about her?"

"She died."

It was the exact middle of the night—the strange, confusing hour that is neither today nor tomorrow, when the zeroes line up on the nursing charts, and outside dark night becomes dark morning, while inside the fluorescent bulbs keep burning their bizarre, timeless energy, reflecting off the linoleum floor.

I found Theresa standing at her mother's bedside, stroking her hair, weeping. She was an African American woman, fortyish, heavyset, in a black tracksuit with pink piping on the sleeves. She wore her hair in tiny braids curled in ringlets around her face, pinned back at the temples with ladybug bobby pins, like a little girl. Her husband, a sinewy man on crutches with a speckle of gray in his beard, hovered quietly in the background. The room was dark; the TV was turned to a choir singing classical music.

The patient looked much like she had when I'd last seen her a few hours earlier, waxy lips parted, thin gray hair combed back from her face. I leaned down to place my stethoscope on her chest and saw the details of her human body up close: the hairs scattered on her upper lip and chin, the black pores on the fleshy tip of her nose, the sticky tears still glistening in the corners of her eyes. On the other side of the stethoscope: a pronounced stillness, the roaring silence I'd never actually heard before. One by one I parted the eyelids and shined my light into the glassy, blank eyes—glimpsing for a moment the depths of the ocean caught in that tiny beam.

When I let go, the eyelids stayed half open. In what seemed like an awkward, clichéd gesture, I pulled them back down with my fingertips, hoping they wouldn't pop open again when I let go, like the eyes of a plastic doll.

Rising, I reached for Theresa's hand and said, "I'm sorry." Then, remembering what I was here to do, I added firmly, "She's died."

Nodding and biting her lip, Theresa whimpered, "One thirty-one."

The time of death.

We were silent for a moment. I held onto her hand. Then abruptly she said, "I need help taking her ring off." Her eyes squeezed tight; her face crumpled. "I don't want to be the one to pull it off her finger."

I thought I saw her husband roll his eyes and shift his weight on his crutches.

In my bravest voice, I offered, "Would you like me to take it off for you?"

She nodded, eyes still closed, head bowed.

I pulled the covers back and gently lifted the thin hand, still warm and alive-feeling. The fingers were curled as though they'd been clutching something—a tissue, a talisman. It occurred to me that it would be a rather morbid picture if, now that I'd volunteered, I could not straighten out the fingers and pull off the ring. I resolved not to be timid. But the fingers were pliable in mine, and I loosened the fist easily. The hand was empty. The ring was a thin gold band topped with a blue stone. With a firm, slow pull and two strong twists, it slid over the knuckle, scraping along with it a thin layer of something slightly wet—dried skin cells maybe, sweat, lotion.

I held the ring out to Theresa, who took it and clasped it to her chest. (Again, I thought, a bit melodramatic.)

"Thank you," she almost whispered. "Thank you for calling me when you did."

Papers to sign, notes to write. Disposition: expired. I went to the stairwell and headed up one flight, my footsteps echoing off the cement walls. I turned to the doorway of the next floor—stopping short, startled.

A locked door: LEVEL 6—ROOF.

I had forgotten that I was already on the highest floor of the hospital. There was nothing else here.

Disconcerted, tired, I turned and hurried back down the stairs. The night went on.

After all those years living apart, there was no time for the life Mo and I wanted so badly to share together. Done with his training (he had specialized in ophthalmology), Mo began practicing independently just as I was starting my intern year. Of course it was hard for him: practicing on his own for the first time, without the guidance of attending physicians or the camaraderie of his co-residents; meeting new people, learning the ropes of a new practice. I saw glimpses of the difficulty, and I was vaguely aware of it. He rubbed his eyes after his long drive home, talked about finding a different job. He operated on Monday mornings, so on Sunday nights he was anxious and irritable; he took a pill to help him fall asleep. When a surgery went badly, he brooded over it for days afterward.

Now I can understand how hard those first few months in practice can be, and I can see that he was carrying his own burdens. But all I could think then was how easy his life was compared to mine. He worked eight to five, Monday through Friday, with weekends off.

A note I wrote in my primary care clinic:

Subjective: 60 y.o. Filipina woman with multiple medical problems, here primarily to discuss a recent upsetting life event: Youngest daughter got pregnant. Patient is very upset, crying a lot. Says multiple times, "Doctor, I want to die." Also expresses desire to kill the father of her daughter's unborn baby, although on further questioning she says she will not do this.

Exam: No acute distress. Tearful.

Assessment and Plan:
Life stressor:
- Discussed at length.
- No suicidal ideation or intent. Patient does not have a specific plan. ("I would not overdose or anything.") Does not own weapon.

Factors preventing her from killing herself:
- Catholic. ("I fear the Lord.")
- Able to contract for safety.
- Declines therapy
- Declines Ativan
- Will return to clinic in 2 weeks before going to Las Vegas to visit her daughter.

The note I wished I could have written:

As soon as I sit down across from her, she bursts into tears. "Doctor, I have some family problem, I'm sorry. I want to talk to you about it." And her face crumples.

I have never met her before.

A petite, pretty Filipina woman with a short, stylish haircut, no makeup, delicate features. A white T-shirt and sweats, freckles scattered across her cheekbones.

It's her daughter—her youngest. Seven months pregnant "by a married man." Her voice breaking again, her shoulders shaking. They learned only a month ago. The daughter managed to keep it hidden until now. (Maybe that's why she took a job in Las Vegas.) It's all a little unclear to me—to the patient, too. She doesn't understand what happened, or how.

"She was a good girl. She is a good girl. She was the one we were counting on."

It is not all about right and wrong, shame and the Church and wedlock. "We were counting on her to take care of us," she explains. "She is R.N. She had a good job here. My husband and me, we are so tired. He has prostate cancer. And he is still working. I am still working. We are both tired of working so hard. My other children, they already have children, so they cannot take care of us. I take care of them, my grandchildren. My oldest daughter has four already. She needs help with the children while she works. She got divorced two years ago. It broke my heart. And now this—I don't know how I can live. My heart is broken again."

This is not all drama and self-pity. Her heart really is broken. She is tired, on the edge. This is a mother who has been caring for her family for forty years, without rest, without relief. And now she has just learned that there will be no one to take care of her. She had imagined, selfishly perhaps— But she has been so selfless! All these years!— that it was nearly her turn to rest, to be taken care of, to be looked after. Instead her daughter is about to produce another baby, another crying helpless life, this time without a father, and she is once again left alone, only giving, only wanting.

She is tired. Oh, she is so tired.

I see my own mother in this woman. I see her fatigue, her weariness. Oh mothers. Poor mothers.

"My husband says, 'Just accept. Just accept.' But I cannot accept, Doctor. In my mind and in my heart—" She presses a tiny fist to her chest, curls herself over it as though to protect her last, precious possession. "I cannot accept. I am angry. I am hurt."

Sometimes she just wants to run away, she says. To leave them all and just be on her own, "whatever may happen."

Yes, I know, I want to tell her. *I want to run away sometimes, too.*

No, I mustn't say that.

Instead I say, "I can tell what a good mother you are. You care tremendously about your family."

"Yes," she says, suddenly clear and firm. "I would do anything to protect them. Anything. Even—" She looks me straight in the eye. "Even I would kill. I would kill that man. That man who did this to my daughter. If we were in the Philippines, he would be dead."

The look in her eye is not one of a faker. I am actually a little bit frightened for him, the father of this unborn child.

I try to make light of it. "Well, now, don't do that," I say, placing my hand on her knee, a gentle, smiling reprimand.

But she does not smile. She does not crack.

I am silent. Finally I say, "Promise me you won't do that."

She shakes her head once. Her hands are trembling. "Anyway I do not have a gun," she says. "And I don't drive. So how can I do it?"

"Well, I'm glad you don't have a gun," I say.

"If I were in the Philippines, I would have him dead," she says again. And I believe her.

As we make a plan to see each other in two weeks, I say to her—because I know it is what I'm supposed to say—"Can you promise me you won't hurt anyone, or yourself, during that time?"

"Yes, I can promise that," she says, frowning. I can tell she is glad I'm taking her seriously. I am glad, too. I am not treading in unthinkable territory, here. This is a passionate human being, a passionate woman. Am I one hundred percent confident that she won't do something terrible in the angriest, most desperate, most painful of moments? No, I am not. And yet I have to let her go. She must go back to her family: her husband with prostate cancer; her daughter, divorced with four children; her other daughter, whom she is afraid she no longer loves, but whom she cannot bear to leave alone, pregnant, in Las Vegas.

She is a mother. A mother of mothers. I cannot hold her back.

SIX WEEKS

DOCTORS COUNT A PREGNANCY in weeks, not months. We know with that level of precision, almost to the day, the stepwise development of the fetus: its organ structures, its sensory perceptions, its nearness to something we call "viability"—the potential to survive outside the womb.

At six weeks, the fetal pole is barely a centimeter in length, a squirming white bean on the ultrasound screen, with a flicker at its center. The beating heart is no more than two rudimentary tubes twisted into a knot, fluttering like wings; the nervous system a vertical ridge running from crown to rump. We measure this "crown-rump length" to date the pregnancy and predict the due date.

Sometimes you see something unexpected. Two squirming white beans: twins. Or, like that woman I saw in prenatal clinic with Dr. K, a fetal pole that looks about six-week size, but instead of wiggling happily away next to its yolk sac, it's just a floating white oval. Like something you might see in a shallow puddle and nudge with your toe. *What is that thing?*

I don't want to use the word "dead," because that implies that there was a life, and strictly speaking, that isn't accurate. Or it isn't what I believe. Nevertheless, the only way I can describe what I saw on the screen that day with Dr. K, what I have seen countless times since, is that it is like the difference between seeing someone asleep and seeing them dead: It is more than just stillness. There is a difference, an absence.

In obstetrics, the technical term for miscarriage is a "spontaneous abortion." It is extremely common in the early weeks of pregnancy, the fate of somewhere between a third and half of all fertilized eggs.

Usually it starts with bleeding. The woman feels something warm in her underwear, or she sees clots in the toilet bowl. She comes to the clinic, tearful and anxious, and we use the ultrasound to look for the embryo and its little flickering heartbeat. If the bleeding continues, there is nothing anyone can do. The uterus, a muscular ball, clamps down with incredible force; the cervix opens; the tiny embryo and the thick, bloody uterine lining are forced out of the body. The pregnancy is over.

If, on the other hand, the heart is still beating and her bleeding stops on its own, everyone is relieved. The pregnancy continues.

Sometimes, like that day in the prenatal clinic, the fetal heartbeat stops, but there is no bleeding. She comes into her doctor's office giddy with expectation after taking a pregnancy test. She learns of the miscarriage only from the ultrasound. This is called a "missed" abortion. In cases like these, the woman has three choices: she may wait for her body to expel the pregnancy, which usually happens in a few days or weeks; she may take medicines to make the uterus cramp, expelling the pregnancy; or she can have an aspiration procedure. This is technically the same procedure as a first-trimester abortion, but instead of terminating the pregnancy, the doctor is only hastening the conclusion of what has already happened.

Removed from the uterus, a six-week embryo is too small to see with the naked eye. In a lab next to the exam room, the doctor rinses away the blood and clots to reveal the gestational sac: a fluff of white cloud floating in a clear plastic dish.

These are hard things to explain to a woman who is naked and crying on the exam table, as I tried to do that morning. "It's not going to become a living baby. It's going to come out of you. You're going to bleed and it's going to fall out."

"But the test," she kept saying. "I'm pregnant. Not bleeding."

"You will bleed soon," I said.

She kept crying and shaking her head. I stood there handing her tissues.

Eventually I asked, "How many children do you have?"

"Three."

I touched her arm. "They're lucky to have you."

When I left the room she was still sitting on the edge of the table, bare-bottomed under the paper drape, sniffling.

After the woman dressed, Dr. K returned to discuss her options with her and schedule a return visit. I moved on to the next patient, who was already waiting in another room.

When I asked Dr. K later what she had decided to do, he told me that she had "some kind of mental disorder," and that she was "not bright."

"I couldn't make her understand expectant management versus a surgical procedure," he said. "I spent so long trying to explain, but she just didn't get it."

My voice caught in my throat. I knew Dr. K had trained at a time when a doctor's expertise was considered far more important than his bedside manner. But when I thought of what had happened in that room, the words he had used, the way he'd stood over her with the probe stuffed in her vagina, I felt sick. It had been like a rape, a violent thing.

The more I think about that patient now, the worse I feel—not just about her interactions with Dr. K. I remember her confused eyes, her broken English. I remember the words I used. I'd tried to choose them carefully, but I had never done this before, and now I realize how easily I could have been misunderstood. "Three kids. Lucky." *This is nothing to cry about. You've already got three. Move on.*

A few weeks later I had my first vacation of residency. Each of us was allowed three weeks off per year, one week at a time.

Mo and I booked a campsite in Capitola for the first week of October. We drove south, stopping at my parents' house in Palo Alto for two nights, where we celebrated my thirtieth birthday. My dad had recently had another stroke, and once again he could hardly move his left arm and leg. He was stumbling around the house, leaning on walls, clutching the furniture.

We arrived late on a Friday night after I finished work. The next morning my mom and I took the dog for a walk. She told me that the day before, she and my dad had driven to the store to pick up groceries for dinner, and afterward he had wanted to stop by the coffee shop. She waited for him in the car. When he came teetering out, coffee in one hand, cane in the other, a young woman came walking down the sidewalk toward him. My mom watched as the woman offered an arm to steady him. "And he yelled at her," Mom said. "Like he always does whenever anyone tries to help him. But it was really awful. He was waving his cane and everything. After he got in the car, I saw her sitting on a bench. She had her head in her hands and she was crying. So I told Dad to wait a second, and I got out and told her, 'I'm sorry. It's not your fault. He does that to everybody.' And she sort of wiped her tears and said, 'It's just that I've been having a bad day.'

"I felt so awful for her," Mom said. Her face crumpled and she started to cry. "It's just so sad. Everyone walks around with these emotions, and then people bump into each other and hurt each other."

I didn't know what to say. I also felt moved by the idea of that young woman—who could have been me, or my sister—crushed by Dad's misdirected anger, his stupid pride. And my heart ached for my mom. I couldn't remember the last time I'd seen her cry.

Later that afternoon, my dad's anger landed on me. I no longer remember the tiny thing that made him explode, his accusations against me. But it crushed me, too, the way it must have crushed that young woman at the coffee shop. It was different, of course, because he's my father, not a stranger. But the feeling was the same: to try to offer someone love and kindness, and to have them respond as though you were trying to hurt them. It was a pain that reached into the very center of me and tore something out. *Am I a monster? What my dad sees in me—is it real?*

Later in the day, I had a moment when I believed that I could put aside that anger and choose compassion instead: compassion for my dad's pain, and his loss, and his fear. I really felt ready to do that. But then Mo and I went for a walk, and he was trying to talk to me about my dad. And all this other, deeper anger began to rise up inside me. It had something to do with the past, and all the times in my life when my dad's response to me had made me hate myself. All the doubts I had about who I was, all the terrible things I sometimes believed about myself—they all seemed to be framed in my dad's accusing stare, the same look he'd given me that afternoon. As though he could see straight past the deceitful surface of loving kindness to the true, selfish, bitter core. *Monster. Monster.*

The next morning when I came downstairs, my dad was wearing an old pair of New Balance sneakers. I hadn't seen him wear anything but his slippers, inside or outside the house, in years. "Dad, where are you going?" I asked, looking pointedly at the sneakers.

He avoided my question. "To the kitchen," he said. Clever.

I knew something was up. Sure enough, later I heard him telling my mom that he had scheduled a driving lesson at 10 a.m.

They had taken away his license that summer, after the third stroke. He was in the process of filing an appeal with the DMV, which would require him to pass a behind-the-wheel driver's test. In order to prepare, he must have registered with the driving school—the same guys who rode around with us when we were fifteen, in the car with the passenger-side brake pedal.

At exactly ten, a corpulent middle-aged guy pulled up in front of the house in a red car with a sign on top. CAUTION: STUDENT DRIVER. He knocked on the front door and asked for Matt. My dad appeared in his sneakers, holding the edge of the couch and lurching forward, one step at a time, making his way toward the friendly (but undoubtedly wary) driving instructor. "How you doin' there, Matt?" the man greeted him. I bolted out the door and went for a walk.

I was barely gone half an hour, but when I arrived back at the house, Dad was already climbing the front steps. The red driving school car was nowhere in sight.

"It's over already?" I asked as I passed him on the stairs.

"It's over," he said.

I paused on the porch and turned. "Well, how did it go?"

"Not very well," he said casually, as though I'd asked him the outcome of a soccer match on TV.

But that casual manner was a front. I knew it mattered to him. He'd put on those sneakers, tied the laces himself. It must have taken him half an hour. He had set up the DMV appointment and the driving lesson. Mom wouldn't have done it for him; she didn't think he should be driving anymore. None of us did.

Later that afternoon, when we were in the car on the way to the campsite, Mo told me, "I don't think your dad's driving lesson worked out."

"What did he tell you?"

"Not much," he said. "Just that at a certain point the instructor dude was like, 'Okay, that's it. It's over. I'm driving you home.'"

"Gosh. I wonder what happened."

"Yeah, he didn't say. Although he did say he was surprised the guy gave him his learner's permit back at the end of it."

"You mean he could have confiscated it?"

"I guess so. The guy told your dad he can still take driving lessons if he wants, just not through that same company."

"Gosh." I remembered how he had cleverly avoided my question that morning. *Dad, where are you going? To the kitchen.* Then on the front porch, the way he said it went *not very well,* when he must have been so bitterly disappointed.

"Oh, Daddy," I whispered.

Mo reached over and patted my hand. "But you know your dad. He was kind of … laughing about it," he said.

But that only made me even more sad.

The next morning I woke up alone in the tent. I lay there a long time before stumbling out into the foggy morning. Mo was scrambling eggs over the campfire. He brought me a mug of tea and I sat at the picnic table, my legs cocooned in my sleeping bag, and opened my diary to write. He said nothing, just put a plate of eggs in front of me and sat next to me with yesterday's newspaper. I wrote until the fog burned away over the ocean below us, thinking I could wake up this way every morning, forever, and I would be happy.

But I had cried the night before as I was falling asleep in the tent on the hard ground. And I'd cried waking up that morning to the sound of the birds and the smell of eucalyptus and wood smoke and the roar of the ocean. I was thinking about my parents.

The way my mom cried when she told me about the woman at the coffee shop; my dad's limp left side, the way he leaned on the furniture, dragging his left foot behind him; and when we left, the way my mom said she wished we could have stayed longer. She had never said that to me before.

A few weeks after that trip, my mother-in-law came over to our house in Martinez bearing an enormous paper bag filled with, as she said, "a few things" for me.

The coming Tuesday was the Hindu ritual day of *Karwa Chauth*. On this day, she explained, Hindu wives in northern India fast from sunrise until moonrise, in order to provide good fortune and good health to their husbands.

"I'm not fasting," I said immediately.

"No, no! You don't fast. You are working too hard for that," she agreed. "Just, there are a few things which you can do."

She began pulling things from the paper bag like a Hindu Mary Poppins: *sindoor* powder for my hair; henna to decorate my hands; little plastic packets filled with mustard seeds, cardamom pods, turmeric, fennel; tea lights; bangles; *ghee*; rose water. Finally, a large metal sieve. In great detail, she explained how each item was to be used in the day's "few rituals." It turned out that this would entail several steps before sunrise (applying the henna to my hands, eating sweets, looking at the stars) and after sunset. The final, most important step was to find the moon at night and view it through the metal sieve.

"Why a sieve?" I asked, holding it up to our kitchen light. It was a cheap tin thing from India, essentially just a shallow dish with holes poked through the bottom. I recognized it as the tool that the women in the village would use to rinse and pick through *daal* before cooking. I could picture them squatting by the spigot or along the river on their strong thighs, talking as they worked. It seemed bizarre that this humble domestic item had found its way into our little home in Martinez, with our brushed-nickel sink and granite countertops and espresso machine.

"It's like a veil, and the moon represents your husband," my mother-in-law said. "Like on your wedding day, you do not look at him directly; you look through the veil. That is the purpose of the sieve."

Memories flashed through my mind as the speckled light hit my face: Mo looking at me through a curtain of white beads that hung from his turbaned forehead; my own neck aching from the weight of the jeweled *dupatta* pinned to my hair; both of us straining to see each other through the heat of the fire and the smoke stinging our eyes.

"Sometimes," she continued, "it is a cloudy night and you cannot see the moon. Then you cannot break the fast until you see it. Then the ladies are very upset."

I raised my eyebrows in mock alarm. "Then what happens?"

She chuckled and leaned over me, placing her hands between my shoulder blades. "Nowadays we just look on the television for the moon. Or we call each other on the phone. You know, my sister in Seattle calls me almost every *Karwa Chauth*, because in Seattle it is cloudy. She cannot see the moon. Or she calls my other sister in L.A. She asks us, 'Do you see the moon? Do you see the moon?' And we tell her, 'Yes, moon is there.' So then she can break her fast."

On *Karwa Chauth*, I completed all the rituals as she'd instructed me—except for the fast. That was too much on a fourteen-hour workday. I got up before five as always, ate a banana before walking up the hill to the hospital, making sure to look at the stars on the way there. It was all partly to humor her, partly to respect her, partly out of some vague superstitious dread that it would be bad luck not to observe these rituals in our very first year of marriage. The first *Karwa Chauth*, she told me, was the most important.

At night, I filled a *thali* with dried fruits, *dhoop*, a small bottle of *ganga* water, and various other auspicious paraphernalia. I smeared *sindoor* in the part of my hair and lit a candle and stepped onto the front porch. The moon was straight ahead in the sky, as though it had been stuck there just for me, as clear and round as the *bindi* on my forehead. I quickly threw the sieve up in front of my eyes and held it there, gazing at the cool, filtered moonlight. Then, unsure of what else to do, I closed my eyes and bowed my head, touching my fingertips to my forehead and my heart as I had learned to do in the temples in India. Then I stepped back inside the house and placed the candle on the kitchen table, to let it burn down to its wick.

"All done?" Mo called from the kitchen.

"I think so."

He emerged holding a pan of glistening pink salmon fillets. "So can I put the fish in the oven? We can eat in ten minutes?"

"Sounds good."

I heard the oven door close and he reemerged, wrapping his arms around my waist. He kissed me on the mouth. "Thanks for doing all that stuff."

"I want to do it."

"It means a lot to my mom."

"We better get your phone and take a picture for her."

"Good idea."

I kissed him back and went to the kitchen to make a salad. The smell of roasting salmon mixed with incense and rose water made me briefly light-headed. But the feeling passed, and I felt the way I did most evenings: tired and hungry.

I had a bizarre dream that night. I was lost somewhere far away, in another country, maybe it was India. I had been told to look for the moon to find my way home. For some reason I was holding a sieve up to the sky, thinking it might help me find the moon. But the sky was black. There wasn't a single star. At first I thought I could see the glow of the moon in the distance, and I walked toward it, clutching the sieve to my eyes. But the farther I walked, the darker the sky became, until there was nothing but black, and I was too scared and tired to walk another step. Then I seemed to be falling into the blackness; it was swallowing me whole, and I was screaming for Mo— trying to scream—but I couldn't make a sound.

Another morning, another prenatal intake, this time with Dr. A, a young, easygoing doctor a few years out of her own residency.

The patient was a twenty-six-year-old G6P2, meaning she'd been pregnant six times, including this pregnancy, and had given birth twice. The other pregnancies had ended in a miscarriage (once) and elective abortions (twice).

The day we saw her, she was eight weeks pregnant by the date of her last menstrual period, but she'd been to the ER the night before, bleeding and cramping. "They told me everything was okay," she said.

"Did they do an ultrasound?" Dr. A asked her.

The patient was a young African American woman with bright eyes, a silver stud through her lip, and a two-year-old son by her side. He was absorbed in a video on her phone. "Uh-huh, they did. But they didn't tell me nothing. They just said I was still pregnant."

"Did you keep bleeding after you left the ER?"

"Yeah, I soaked through a pad," she said.

Dr. A flicked a switch on the ultrasound machine and it hummed to life. She continued with her questions. "Is this a planned pregnancy? Do you think you're going to keep it?"

The woman propped herself on her elbows and tilted her head. "We didn't plan on it," she said. She gave a coy smile, tilting her head the other way, rolling her eyes a little. "I don't know. I might keep it. I might not. I don't know."

"Well, let's just do the ultrasound and see what we're dealing with," Dr. A said.

As Dr. A coated the vaginal probe with gel, the woman lay down on the table. She kept musing out loud about the pregnancy and what she was going to do about it. "I already got a lot of work with just him and his sister," she said, gesturing to her little boy, who had dropped the phone and was trying to climb onto her lap. Dr. A inserted the probe and found the pregnancy, a seven-week fetal pole with a clear flicker at its center. The young woman asked to see the image; she pulled her son onto the table with her and pointed at the screen. "Look, baby!" She cooed. "There's the heartbeat! You see it? You see the heart?"

The little boy glanced at the screen, then scrambled to the floor again to find the phone.

Dr. A pointed to a dark fluid collection next to the gestational sac that looked like blood (called a subchorionic hemorrhage). "Harmless," she said. "But it might be the cause of your bleeding. Sometimes we see that. It might also be an early miscarriage. Only time will tell us."

The patient squinted at the image and said, "Is there any way this could be twins? Because the daddy is a twin."

"Hmm," Dr. A said. "You know ..." She moved the probe back and forth and leaned into the screen. "There's no way to tell for sure, but actually I would say yes, it's also possible that there was a second pregnancy there, and that that fluid is all that remains of it. Maybe your bleeding last night was you passing the other pregnancy."

"Oh my gosh!" the patient squealed.

"But it's important to understand that even if there was a twin, it isn't there anymore. And it's still possible that you might lose this pregnancy as well, since you're still bleeding."

The patient said she understood, but the new light in her eyes betrayed her excitement.

Dr. A finished the ultrasound, removed the probe, and asked her how she wanted to proceed.

Again the patient squinted and said, "I don't know …" Then looking beyond us to the wall, she added, "The dad, he don't believe in abortion." She gestured toward her son. "That's how come I had him."

"Does the father know about this pregnancy?" Dr. A asked.

"Oh yeah, he knows. That's why—Honestly I'm probably just gonna end up having it." She looked past us again, that same coy smile playing on her lips. "Yup. I am. I'm gonna do it. I'm gonna have another baby!" Finally she looked straight at us. She was beaming.

I was horrified. I had never seen a woman make a decision like this right before my eyes. It was not the decision I had expected, or wanted for her. I wanted to shake her by the shoulders and say, "You do realize, this is not just about how you feel this moment, today. This is about your body, a forty-week pregnancy, and then the rest of your life. A third child. How will you cope? How will you afford it? Think about this." I thought Dr. A should have said something to try to guide her, remind her of these things. But Dr. A just said, "Okay then, great." She handed her a wad of tissue to wipe off the gel and went to book another appointment for her.

That afternoon before falling asleep, I sat up in bed, writing about the young woman and her pregnancy. I thought about her "decision" (if that's what you could even call it, I mused bitterly) and wondered whether and how we had failed her.

Dr. A, I decided, should have been more careful about showing her the ultrasound, because the woman seemed to have been influenced by the image of the fetal heartbeat, the idea of having possibly conceived twins—even if only one remained. That and the fact that the father didn't "believe in abortion." I shook my head, scribbling furiously, all the while neglecting to consider how I might have felt differently if she had been a white woman in her thirties, well-educated, articulate—a woman more like me.

She was wrong, I thought. She had chosen the path of least resistance, the apparently "easy" thing to do: stay pregnant. Everyone will be happy for you. No one can question you. No one can call you a murderer. No one can tell you you'll regret it, even if, maybe, you will.

I remembered all the women in the abortion clinic in medical school—black, white, rich, poor—how scared and vulnerable they'd seemed. But they were the brave ones, I thought. Even though they might have been cast as heartless murderers or careless girls or helpless victims, these were the women with perhaps the greatest sense of control and agency over their own lives, because they had chosen the demonized option of abortion; they had stuck to that decision; they'd done their research and found their way to the abortion clinic.

This woman, I felt sorry for her, but I couldn't relate to her. In a way, I thought, I could relate more to the abortion patients. At least they'd made an actual decision. At least they'd done something.

My empathy in those early years was crude, if well intentioned. My understanding of "choice" was limited to the choices I'd made, choices of privilege and control. There was a lot I didn't know.

Outside of residency, at the edges of my daily existence, life went on. My dad kept having strokes; I feared he might not live much longer. My mom seemed at a breaking point, caring for him alone.

My relationship with Mo's parents, meanwhile, became more fraught. Whenever I had a day off, it seemed like they always wanted to see us. "Can't you get together with them without me?" I whined.

One afternoon in Sacramento, Mo's mom pressured us playfully about when we were going to have children. My whole body flashed with anger; I gritted my teeth and left the room, not wanting to make a scene, not trusting myself to stay calm.

Afterward I said to Mo, "You have to tell your mom that she can never, ever ask us about having kids ever again. That is private. It is none of her business."

He just nodded, stone-faced. "Okay," he said. "I'll tell her."

The next time they called asking to see us, I told Mo I wanted to stay home.

When he came back after a short dinner with them at a nearby restaurant, I asked him how it had gone. "It was fine," he said. "They asked about you, of course. I told them you were working."

I was furious. "Why did you have to lie? Why couldn't you just tell them it's my one day off and I had other things to do?"

He shook his head. "I didn't want to give them a reason ..."

"A reason to what?"

"A reason not to like you."

There was hardly ever time to write. Even when I got home from the hospital before dark, I was too tired to put my thoughts into words. Mo said, "Don't worry, you'll write tomorrow." But he didn't understand. Writing wasn't something that needed to happen just now and then, at some time or another. *Every day,* I thought frantically. *It should be every day. Otherwise I'll lose it. I am losing it.*

Sometimes when I left the hospital after working all night, or when I was just passing an hour until it was time to go back in again, I would walk down to the water, on the path that wound along the edge of the bay under a bowl of golden hills. As I walked, I turned the same questions over and over in my mind, questions that had plagued me since medical school. Could I leave? Was it too late?

I had long believed that regret was a choice, something I could decide to either harbor or release. But the deeper I got, the more I began to see how regret could be something real, permanent.

Now that residency is behind me and I'm doing the work I was meant to do—work I love and am good at—I feel I made a narrow escape. I almost gave it up, almost lost my chance at this. But at the time, all I could think about was getting out.

Today before leaving work, I called Kat, the ultrasound technician, into one of the exam rooms and asked her to close the door. "Can you do me a favor? If you're not comfortable, you can say no."

I had turned on the ultrasound machine, which sat humming in the corner next to the exam table. The vaginal probe was already coated in gel.

"Sure," Kat said. "Of course."

I shimmied out of my scrub pants and lay on the table, hoisting my feet into the footrests. She pressed the probe into me with her deft, gentle touch, as I'd seen her do for a thousand patients. The gel on the tip of the probe coated my pubic hair and then my insides, cold and slimy. A shiver ran from my belly button to my toes.

I turned my head toward the screen and waited for the familiar image to appear: gray oval in a flashlight beam, black gestational sac. And in the middle of the sac, there it was: my tiny white bean.

I propped myself on my elbows, leaning toward the screen. I glanced at Kat. "Is that …?"

"Yeah," she said. "Can't you see it?" She zoomed in on the unmistakable flicker: the heartbeat.

I said, "Does the heartbeat seem kind of … weak to you?"

"What do you mean, 'weak?'" She said it curiously, as though I were teaching her some academic distinction.

"I mean, I don't know—the heartbeat just looks sort of … weak."

She hesitated, then looked straight at me. "I don't know, Dr. Henneberg. All they taught us in ultrasound tech school is that cardiac activity is either 'present' or 'absent.' We didn't learn about 'strong' or 'weak' or anything like that. Is that a thing?"

I let my shoulders drop back on the table and gave a little laugh. "No," I said. "You're totally right, Kat. It's not a thing. I'm just being … I don't know what. I'm just being nervous."

She nodded. "Do you want me to measure it?"

"Would you, please?"

She scanned the probe in an arc inside of me, side to side, front to back, until she had the best possible image. Then she clicked, drew a line straight through the middle of the embryo—the crown-rump length— and read the number to me.

"So," I said. "About six weeks."

"Six weeks and four days," she said. Then she eased the probe out of my body.

"Thanks." I stood up, drawing the paper drape through my legs and using it to wipe off the ultrasound gel in one motion, acting the part of the experienced patient.

"No problem," Kat said. "Can I ask, is this ... I mean ... were you trying?"

"Yeah," I said. "We've been trying for a few months. And what do you know? It worked."

TWELVE WEEKS

ONE MORNING ON MY hospital rounds, shortly after our camping trip and *Karwa Chauth*, a patient told me, "You're the best doctor I've ever had!" I had met him only the day before, and I'd hardly done anything but talk with him. He was a big, broad-chested man in his fifties with chronic obstructive pulmonary disease and right-sided heart failure. The kind cardiologist, who loved teaching residents, told me the man had a "great exam," but when I listened that morning I could barely hear his heart beating through the wide, hollow barrel of his chest. I just pressed my stethoscope to his ribs and nodded.

Afterward, as I squatted by the head of his bed to explain the diuretics we were giving him and how important it was he keep taking them at home, he told me I was a great doctor. "I appreciate how you don't just stand there; you get down by my side and talk to me. None of the others do that."

I remembered once when my dad came in for a burger at the Palo Alto Creamery, a diner where I worked during summers in college. It was a busy lunch hour and he wasn't seated in my section, but things slowed down as he was finishing his meal, and I stopped by his booth. "I've been watching you," he said. "I notice how you crouch down beside the people and meet them at their level. That is good. You don't talk down to them, you talk to them eye to eye."

At the time I was annoyed with him for pointing this out with his air of approval, as though he were my supervisor giving me feedback on my performance, as though I wasn't a good waitress unless he told me so. He could just as easily have found something to criticize, and I would have felt bad about myself the rest of the day.

After I graduated from college and Dad had his first stroke, I spent the rest of the year living at home with my parents, waitressing at the Creamery. My dad and I fought bitterly, especially when my mom was away. One afternoon (Mom was on a work project in Cambodia), I was heading out the door on my way to the Creamery, and suddenly we were fighting about something—I can't remember what, but he was yelling at me, and I was yelling back at him, telling him he didn't know anything and he couldn't tell me what to do. His face was taut and red, all the tendons in his neck and arms standing out like wires. It was the angriest I'd seen him since the stroke.

Suddenly he seemed to lose control of his body. His left arm and leg, which had regained most of their strength over a few months, twisted and tightened inward, and he collapsed to the floor. Even as he was falling, he kept yelling. As he lay there, his left arm and leg twitching and jerking at his side like a sick animal, he spat out, "Look what you did! You gave me another stroke! Get out of this house! Get out of here!" And I did. I left him there on the floor. I ran.

This was before I knew any medicine. In residency, I would learn the term "recrudescence," a phenomenon in which a person with residual weakness from a stroke loses strength in the same area, temporarily, during periods of physical or psychological stress. Of course I didn't know this at the time. But I knew enough to understand that I hadn't "given" my dad another stroke. I knew it was the anger that had caused him to fall down. Dad's anger always had been, and was still, a powerful thing, an almost physical force.

Nevertheless, I was terrified.

A few blocks away I stopped, gasping and crying. Standing on the sidewalk, I called my aunt Margaret and told her what had happened. I asked if she thought I should try to reach my mom in Cambodia and ask her to come home. "Chrissy, your mom didn't get on a plane to Germany when your dad had his stroke," she said. "I don't think she's going to get on a plane now."

So I went to work.

My dad was right: I was a good waitress. I liked to squat beside customers while I answered their questions and took their orders. I always wore the same pair of jeans when I worked, and I remember exactly how they felt sliding against my thighs, the tug of my apron across my lap and its strings pressing into the small of my back. Sometimes the customers would tell me, "You're great at what you do," or "You have a beautiful smile," and I would glow inside.

I glowed inside when that patient complimented me. It reminded me of what my dad had said that day. And instead of feeling annoyed, I wanted to call him right then and tell him, "Daddy! You were right! You were right!"

Even after his subsequent strokes, Dad managed to stay at home by himself when Mom traveled, with a caretaker coming in the mornings to help him bathe, shave, and prepare lunch. During residency, whenever Mom was away and I had a day off, I would drive down to keep him company.

One day I arrived in the middle of the afternoon after sleeping as late as I could. I made coffee and brought it to him in his study, where he sat in his red armchair. We sat talking in the afternoon sunlight that slanted through the French doors. I didn't tell him anything about work or the hospital. He didn't ask. He talked about his new hearing aids, the birthday present he'd bought for Mom online, his blood pressure medications. After half an hour I said I wanted to run some errands. I knew he didn't expect me to spend the whole afternoon with him. It was enough just to be there, another warm body moving through the empty house. I walked to the store and bought salmon and bok choy for dinner. On my way home I got a text from Mo. He said he'd had two "bad cases" while he was operating that morning. I told him I was in Palo Alto. He asked if I wouldn't mind coming home a little early.

Mo rarely asked me to do anything for him. I told him of course I would come.

I cooked an early dinner for myself and my dad; neither of us said much while we ate. I cleaned up the kitchen, packed the leftovers, drove back to Martinez and reheated dinner for Mo. We sat on the couch. I asked him questions about the surgeries, but he didn't explain the details. I didn't understand exactly what had gone wrong. I felt more sorry for him than for the patients; I didn't care much about their cataracts. But I was glad, even relieved, that he had asked me to come home. I was glad that what he needed to feel better was to be with me.

When I returned to the hospital after a few days off for Thanksgiving, my service was filled with new patients. One stood out as an unusual case: Denise Winters, a thirty-six-year-old woman with metastatic colon cancer. According to the chart, she had undergone open abdominal surgery four days earlier and was sent to the surgical floor to recover. Over the weekend she had developed difficulty breathing and was transferred to the step-down unit, where she could receive supplemental oxygen and closer monitoring. A chest X-ray showed a pneumonia; sputum cultures were growing *Pseudomonas*—drug-resistant bacteria.

"Hey, who the hell is this lady?" I asked Ruth, another intern. She was working at the computer next to mine, and she had covered my service for much of the past week. "Thirty-six-year-old with colon cancer? Now she has a Pseudomonal pneumonia?"

She leaned over my shoulder to look at the screen. "Oh, shit. I forgot to tell you about her. Denise Winters. She's a really sad case. Severe developmental delay from birth, blind, maybe some cerebral palsy. Can't talk, can't walk. G-tube. Totally dependent on her parents. Children's Hospital type of patient, you know?"

She was referring to the kids we had all cared for on our pediatrics rotations in medical school: children with severe developmental diseases, cerebral palsy, rare genetic disorders, who spent most of their lives at Children's Hospital (Oakland, Philadelphia, Houston, wherever) with one problem after another, including feeding difficulties, pneumonias, other infections. Few of these children survived into adulthood. Apparently Denise Winters had.

"And now she has colon cancer at thirty-six?" I said. "God, that sucks. Is it genetic?" Certain gene mutations could be passed through families causing multiple polyps and early colon cancers. Usually a parent or sibling would have been stricken with cancer at a young age as well.

Ruth shrugged. "I met her for the first time post-op. She was working pretty hard to breathe yesterday. I didn't deal with much else except getting the X-ray and transferring her. Her mom is a real nice lady, though. She's at the bedside 24-7—you know the type. I'm sure she can tell you everything there is to know."

When I approached the room, the sliding glass door was shut. The sea-foam green curtain behind it was left open a crack so the nurse could see the telemetry screen above the bed.

Peering into the dark room, I saw the blue number on the screen: 90%. Her oxygen saturation—fair, not great. Beside that was a wavy line showing the rise and fall of her breathing. The waveform was steady, but the rate, thirty-two breaths per minute, was fast. Not the slow, rolling rhythm of ocean waves on a wide beach, but the quick licks of water at a lake's edge.

Beneath the glow of the screen, a dark form under a blanket took up most of the bed. It looked like a great sea lion, its bulk rising and falling with each breath. Surrounding it on the bed were several smaller lumps, difficult to make out in the dark, but they appeared to be piles of blankets.

Beside the bed, also draped with a blanket, was a second form. This one was distinctly human, even classical, perched there on the edge of an armchair: the curve of the shoulders, the angle of the neck, the drape of the limbs over the guardrail. Instantly recognizable, even in the dark: a mother keeping vigil over her child.

I slid the door open. "Good morning," I whispered. "Sorry it's early."

Mrs. Winters looked up, her tired face instantly alert when she saw my white coat, scrubs, and badge.

I saw it in her eyes: I was the first doctor she'd seen today. All the questions and worries of the long night lay stored up for me.

The figure in the bed emitted a deep groan but did not budge.

I stepped inside and introduced myself as I always did: "Dr. Chris Henneberg—please call me Chris." Mrs. Winters stood and shook my hand. She was a petite, buxom woman with bright blue eyes and perfectly white, straight teeth. Her skin was fair and smooth; her white hair was cut in a pixie that was growing over the tops of her ears. Her fingernails were short, bitten; the cuticles were neat half-moons. "Liz Winters, Denise's mom. It's nice to meet you, Chris. You're the intern, is that right?"

Her tone was kind, reserved but not patronizing. This was a woman who knew hospitals; she had probably spent much of her life in rooms like this one. She understood that today was a new day, the Monday after a holiday weekend, and that a new "team" of doctors would be taking over the care of her daughter. In the wee hours of the morning, she must have spoken with the nurses, gathering our names and titles. She also knew that not all doctors were created equal. As an intern, I was at the bottom of the doctors' hierarchy, but I still held some nominal power within the hospital machine. I would not be the doctor making decisions or giving final answers, but I could perhaps serve as a source of information and a messenger to the attending surgeon and the nurses. I could be of some use to her.

I sometimes think this is the greatest bond between an intern and patients and their families. They want so badly to believe that someone will help them. And I wanted so badly to believe I could help.

"Yes," I said. "I'm the intern. I was away last week, but I'll be here every day now. How is Denise doing?"

"Oh Chris." She said my name as though we'd known each other for years. But she was not manipulative or cloying. She had put her trust in me already. "She's not doing well at all. She's in pain. She's really in pain. And her breathing, it's still awful."

Closer to the bed, now, I could hear that Denise's breaths were not just rapid, they were raspy and labored. "Has her breathing gotten any better during the night? Or worse?"

"Oh, definitely better," she said. "It's much better since they put her on the oxygen. I just can't stand to listen to it. She hasn't had a pneumonia in years. I'd forgotten how awful it sounds."

I turned to the huge form under the blanket. "Denise?" I said, flipping on the light over the bed. Her eyes were open, but they were unseeing pearls. She did not turn her head toward my voice. She looked straight through me with the unmistakable, empty gaze of the congenitally blind.

I turned back to her mother, unsure what to say next. I had already read the operative report. The attending surgeon, Dr. W, had opened Denise's abdomen in hopes of removing the bulk of the tumor, but what he found was worse than expected: tumor everywhere, blossoming out of the length of her colon; studding the wall of the abdomen, the kidneys; budding in the liver like cauliflower. He had sewn her right back up. There was nothing to do, nothing to cut out that would make the slightest bit of difference. Her fate, like her abdominal wall, was sealed. It was only a matter of time.

Looking down at her, I understood that the pneumonia was the least of Denise's problems. But I had the feeling no one had told this to her mother. Liz Winters was worried about the pneumonia; she seemed to think the cancer was gone.

It was not my job to break the news to her. Dr. W should have told her, days ago. But he would be furious if I tread on that sacred ground. For now my job was to examine Denise: assess her breathing, her wound, her pain, then report back to Dr. W with my findings.

I had no idea where to begin.

I remembered Children's Hospital. Many of the patients there had been too young, too sick, or too cognitively impaired to communicate. "Veterinary medicine," some doctors called it. You couldn't ask them where they hurt, whether the pain was getting better or worse. It was the parents who answered the questions, usually the mother. She knew. She was the expert. From hours, days, years spent observing patterns and interpreting the sounds of her wordless, helpless child. She could tell you where it hurt.

Denise coughed a wet-sounding cough that racked her whole body, followed by a thick, raw moan, like a barn animal. "That's it," her mother said. "That moaning sound. That's not like her. Something is hurting her. Every time she coughs. But I don't know—is it the cough that hurts in her chest? Or is it because the cough shakes her belly?" She reached across the bed, making slight adjustments to the blankets around Denise's body. I could see now that these piles of blankets had been carefully arranged by a mother's hand, each one strategically placed to brace Denise's body against her tremulous coughing spells, to try to lessen her pain.

I watched. Then I asked, "Is it okay if I examine her?"

She nodded. "Yes, of course."

I pulled back the sheet, exposing the white, rubbery expanse of Denise's abdomen, the train track of her stapled incision coursing vertically from sternum to pubic bone, making a c-shaped detour around her navel, like a traffic circle. Her belly was still swollen with air from the operation and, most likely, with the fluid being released from her massive tumors.

I inspected the incision for signs of infection, pressing gently around the edges with my fingertips. When I tried to press deeper, she moaned and batted my hand away. I listened to her heart and lungs, then straightened and tucked my stethoscope into my pocket.

I explained that sputum cultures were now growing *Pseudomonas*. The weekend team had chosen the right antibiotics for the pneumonia, and we would continue these for now. They seemed to be working, since Denise's oxygen saturation was consistently above ninety percent. Her incision also looked good to me. No redness or pus, no signs of infection. "And I'll be back with Dr. W later this morning to see her again," I said.

I expected Mrs. Winters to press me for more details or decisions, but she did not. She knew better than to waste time grilling the intern. "Thank you, Chris," she said. "I really appreciate your taking care of Denise."

I told her to have the nurse page me with any questions, then I left the room.

On rounds that morning, huddled in an office on the med-surg floor with Dr. W, I presented my findings, focusing on Denise's breathing trouble and cough. "From a surgical standpoint, she's recovering well," I said. "I think the pneumonia is her most, ah, urgent clinical problem."

"Mmm-hmm. I agree." He did not look up.

I wondered when he would raise the main issue: the inoperable cancer, the fatal prognosis for this young woman. He was silent, then glanced at me and said, "Good, so, you'll continue the current antibiotics and proceed with routine post-operative care. Anything else on her?"

I paused. "Just one thing. I, ah … I read the operative report."

He lowered his chin and looked at me. "Congratulations. I expect you to read the op report for all the surgical patients under your care."

"Right. Of course. I just—I thought maybe someone should tell the mother about the findings, you know, explain the significance. I think—I mean I'm pretty sure she doesn't know. The prognosis."

Dr. W put down his pen and leaned back in his chair. "Oh, you're pretty sure about that, are you?"

"I—"

"Dr. Henneberg, do you think I'm a good surgeon?"

"Yes, sir," I answered.

"Do you think that I would ever walk out of an operating room where I've just opened up the patient's abdomen to remove a cancer, where the patient's mother is waiting in the lobby, sick with worry, and that I would not make it my first task to find that mother and tell her the outcome of the surgery to the best level of detail that she can possibly understand and absorb?"

"No, I don't think that. It's just that, well, she seemed like she didn't know, or didn't understand—"

"Do you think I would let—what day is it now, Monday? Do you think I would let four days go by without making sure the patient and the family understand the outcome of a surgery like this one, and its implications?"

"No, I just—"

"What exactly was your concern, Dr. Henneberg?"

My face burned. I said, "I'm sorry, Dr. W. This morning when I talked to the patient's mother, it seemed like she didn't know. She seemed really focused on the pneumonia, like she didn't even know that the cancer was, ah, inoperable. Terminal."

"I see." We sat there for a moment. "Do you have children?" he asked.

I swallowed. "No. Not yet."

"Well. Then try to remember what I'm about to tell you. When or if you ever become a mother, then I think you will understand it: there's a little something called denial. It can be a very, very powerful thing. Especially for parents. Especially for mothers. Even for mothers who have been through a lot, like the mother of this particular patient, who has endured a tremendous amount of suffering."

I stared at him. He continued. "I seem to remember that you take a particular interest in women's health? Obstetrics? Is that right?"

I felt tears beginning to rise up behind my eyes. I nodded.

"When you take care of thousands of mothers, as I have, you eventually see a lot of bad things happen, a lot of mothers who have to accept bad things happening to their babies, their children. But nothing will bring it home for you like being a parent yourself. Do you understand what I'm getting at?"

I nodded again. My heart thudded in the base of my throat. The hum of the computers in the office seemed to grow louder, roaring and vibrating in my ears.

"Denial, Dr. Henneberg. That mother, Mrs. Winters—she knows exactly what I found in her daughter's abdomen. I went over it with her multiple times to make sure she understood. I'm not a counselor or a social worker, but I got those people involved right away. I made sure they knew to talk to the family about palliative care, about hospice. She's heard the whole thing. She's no dummy. If she's focusing on the pneumonia, that's her choice to focus on the pneumonia. It's not my job as the surgeon to psychologize her until she can overcome denial and reach a point of acceptance. But it's my job to tell her what I found in her daughter's abdomen and to make sure she understands those findings, and you'd better believe I did that. So I want you to be careful about the assumptions you make. I'd like you to assume, as your default, that I am doing my job as a surgeon. That is, of course, unless I give you reason to think otherwise. Is that a reasonable request?"

"Yes, Dr. W. I'm sorry."

"Fine. Apology absolutely accepted. Let's move on to the next patient, shall we?"

Dr. W and I visited Denise together later that morning. We spoke at length with her mother. One of the first things she said to Dr. W was that her husband had spoken with the hospice representatives that morning, and someone from the agency would be coming to meet with them at the hospital later in the week. She spoke with a steady voice and met Dr. W's gaze with brave eyes. "I think that's wise," he said. "To have hospice involved early. Thank you for updating me. It helps me to take the best possible care of Denise. We are focused on details here in the hospital; that's our job. So it is helpful to know that you, and the hospice team, have the big picture in mind." Liz Winters' eyes brimmed with tears, but they did not spill.

I scolded myself. I understood now: the reason Liz Winters hadn't spoken of Denise's prognosis that morning wasn't because she couldn't handle it. It was because she thought I couldn't handle it. Maybe I couldn't.

Dr. W examined Denise almost exactly as I had. He listened to her heart and lungs, traced every centimeter of the incision with his eyes, then with a gloved fingertip. He touched her abdomen even more gently than I had, nudging it with his fingertips, as though he were tipping a tiny rocking horse, back and forth, back and forth.

While I was writing my notes in the afternoon, I remembered one more question I'd forgotten to ask. I returned to Denise's room a third time.

She was sleeping, finally. Liz was curled up with a book in the armchair.

"There's something I forgot to ask you," I said to Liz. "It's about, ah, the family history. You probably already know this but colon cancer is quite rare in someone Denise's age. Sometimes it can be due to gene mutations that are carried in families …"

I stopped. Liz was looking straight at me, shaking her head resolutely from side to side.

I thought of what Dr. W had said. Denial. "So … there's no family history?"

"No, I'm afraid not," Liz said. "Quite literally, none. We adopted her when she was an infant."

Adopted.

Whatever disbelieving look was on my face, Liz Winters had encountered it a thousand times before. But she did not sigh or act annoyed at having to explain herself to me. "It was very important to me. It was something I always wanted to do. I had polio when I was a kid. And the doctors told my mom I would never walk again. But she was so devoted to me. She spent hours with me every day, training me, moving my legs and my arms. She did it all herself, the doctors didn't help her at all. And so I always felt like ...like this was something I wanted to do. It's my way of repaying my mother, because I could never repay her. If that makes sense."

I nodded. "I think so. Yeah, I understand." But I did not. I did not understand.

Liz Winters went on: "Tom was against it at first—the adoption. We're Mormons. It's not ... typical in our community. Especially for a young couple without children of their own. But he came around. He knew how important this was to me. And now, of course, he can't imagine our lives without her. I spend so much time with her, just the two of us. She's more than a daughter to me. She's my best friend." She gave a little laugh, just a push of breath. "I tell her she's my soul mate."

Her words brought me back to myself, and to Dr. W's question that morning: do you have children? And my answer: not yet.

I had always thought I would be a mother. Not because I imagined motherhood as something I would enjoy or even be particularly good at—the opposite, in fact. I believed I was too selfish, too focused on my own needs, to ever be a great mom.

Perhaps if I had married someone else more like me, a little more selfish, driven by his own needs and ambitions, I might have talked myself out of motherhood altogether. But that was not the person I'd married. In Mo's parents' world, and in his world too, the whole point of marriage was to have children, to grow the family. To deviate from that would be the worst possible thing I could do to him, or to them. It was not that I felt my hand was forced. It was just that I knew I had given up that option, the option of childlessness, when I married Mo. Motherhood was in my future, whether I was looking forward to it or not.

But since entering residency, that future was beginning to feel more real, more frightening. I was thirty—not old, I knew—but I still had two and a half more years of residency to go. From what I'd heard about raising an infant, it sounded as if I would be signing up for residency all over again: long days and sleepless nights, no time for myself, hardly time to eat or go to the bathroom. I could not imagine feeling ready for that anytime soon. Perhaps ever. And all of that was the best-case scenario: a healthy baby, my own baby. To choose motherhood seemed like an enormous sacrifice. To choose what Liz Winters had chosen—to raise another woman's baby, a child who would never walk or talk, never look into her eyes and tell her, "Mommy, I love you"—I did not understand it.

And yet here they were. And the love between them—it pulsed in the room like an electric field. It was a love more pure than anything I had ever seen.

"Do you mind if I asked how old you were? When you ... became her mom?"

"I don't mind," she said. "I was twenty-two."

"Do you have other children?" I asked.

"No. No other children." She put her hand on top of Denise's, where it rested on a pillow, and stroked the swollen blue patch of skin where an IV had been. "We never even tried. She is enough."

Denise did make a complete recovery from her pneumonia and her surgery. Two days later she was out of the step-down unit and back on the med-surg floor, where she remained for nearly two weeks. I dreaded going to her room every day, hearing her moan in pain, seeing her flap her hands against the mattress and wave her head from side to side, her eyes wide and burning.

None of this fazed her mother. I never saw Liz leave Denise's bedside. Denise's father, Tom, came and went during the day, returning home to sleep. But Liz was there every morning when I arrived, curled in the armchair under a blanket, sometimes half-asleep, but always there. "I've never spent a night away from her," she told me.

CHRISTINE HENNEBERG

As Denise recovered, I saw another side of her emerge. I saw her smile—never at me, but often at Liz. I saw her laugh. I saw her shout in protest when something didn't go her way: when her father left in the evening, or when her mother insisted on giving her a sponge bath.

Liz knew the meaning of her daughter's every grimace, every tilt of her chin, every moan or grunt or occasional bleat of laughter. She did not dote on her, as I thought some Children's Hospital parents did with their kids. In some ways she treated her like the grown woman she was. When I was explaining the latest test or X-ray result and Denise burst out in a high-pitched moan, trying to get her mother's attention, Liz turned to her and said, "Denise, Chris is talking to me. Wait your turn, please." And Denise smacked her lips and waited. She seemed to understand.

Maybe their relationship was not particularly unique. Maybe I was just seeing it more intimately and with less judgment because of the person I knew Liz to be, the choice she had made.

As the day approached for Denise's discharge, I began to feel sorry that she was leaving—or rather, sorry to say goodbye to Liz. The hospice agency had arranged to take over Denise's care when they returned home. A hospital bed had been ordered; a nurse was due to visit every other day. Dr. W predicted "a few months, maybe several months," for Denise to live. She would be at home, surrounded by familiar objects and faces and routines. Still, my heart ached at the thought of Liz losing her daughter, her dear companion, her soul mate.

On the day of Denise's discharge, I said to Liz Winters what I sometimes said to patients I'd grown fond of during a long hospital stay: "Selfishly, I'm sorry you guys won't be here anymore to brighten my morning. But of course I'm glad Denise can leave the hospital now, and I hope she doesn't have to come back here again."

Liz's eyes filled with tears, and she looked away from me. I realized immediately that I had said the wrong thing: *I hope she doesn't have to come back here again.* Denise's life—and much of Liz's life—had been lived in the hospital. That vigil Liz kept every night, curled beside her daughter's bed, was the site of her deepest care and love for her daughter. Denise might have months left to live, but part of Liz had already died that morning, the minute she stretched her aching limbs and stood up from that armchair in the pre-dawn, fluorescent hospital light. They were going home.

She wiped the back of her hand across her eyes and placed her palm on Denise's hair. Denise tilted her head back, pressing her face into her mother's hand.

"Oh Chris," Liz said, and her voice reminded me of the day I had first met her, as though she'd been just waiting to pour her heart out to me. "It's the best and the worst thing in the world, you know. To be needed."

Christmas Eve.

I was hoping the last patient on my clinic schedule wouldn't show up, but there she was. I'd met her a few times already in my six months as her doctor. She was a sixty-seven-year-old Indian woman who normally came with her husband and grown daughter. Usually her daughter translated for her from their native Malayalam. They were Christians, from the Indian state of Kerala.

This time she came alone—straight from work, she explained in her broken English.

She had well-controlled diabetes and rather refractory Parkinson's disease, a condition that more often strikes men, but she was unlucky. She worked in the kitchen at an Indian restaurant, where her pronounced tremor made it hard for her to perform many of her duties. She also suffered from low back pain—another problem at work, where she stood on her feet for hours at a time. She explained she had no choice but to remain at this job for as long as they would keep her. At her age, with her limited English, it would be hard to find anything else, and she was the sole breadwinner for her family. Her husband (also my patient) had gone blind last year from complications of diabetes. One of their daughters was studying to be a nurse, but she didn't yet have her California nursing license; their other daughter had just had a baby and was living in their home.

None of these details had come up in prior visits with her daughter translating. Only today, alone, did she begin to paint the whole picture for me: the shaking was so bad it kept her awake at night. "Whole body is shaking, even brain is shaking. No rest. Medicines not helping." She told me how she woke up at 3 a.m. every day and prayed for one hour. After that she walked to the bus stop, took a bus to the train station, and then took the train to the restaurant in San Francisco, where she trembled and her back hurt—especially when she had to lift heavy pots of water. Then in the evening, she took the train back to the bus again.

"The situation is very difficult," she said. She sat straight-backed, her face flat, almost blank. Her hands, resting on her knees, trembled in that classic Parkinsonian way, as though she were rolling strips of tissue paper between her fingers. "But it is no problem, Doctor. God is good. He will help me." Her face softened and she began to cry.

I had her sit on the exam table and asked her to unzip her jacket. It was a worn yellow fleece with "SAN FRANCISCO" and the Golden Gate Bridge embroidered over the breast pocket, the kind they sold at the airport. Underneath she wore a traditional *salwar kameez,* a flowing cotton tunic over billowing pants. Her gray hair was combed flat across the top of her head, pulled back into a tight bun.

I placed my stethoscope on her chest and listened to her heart and lungs. I wanted her to feel cared for, to feel that I was doing something for her.

I asked her when she would have her next appointment with the neurologist. Two weeks. Then I told her gently—in case the neurologist hadn't, or wouldn't—that sometimes the medicines we have for Parkinson's work well, but sometimes they don't. "I'm sorry I'm not able to do more to help," I said.

She shook her head, a deferential wag from ear to ear. "It's no problem, Doctor. God is good. He will help me." I sensed she was trying to comfort me, assuage my guilt. But I also sensed the harsh accusation against me, against all of us, against the path I'd chosen. *Don't worry, Doctor. God will help me, since you cannot.*

I am twelve weeks pregnant now—nearly at the end of the first trimester. I've come down to Palo Alto for a night to visit my dad. Mom is out of the country for two weeks. I know he'll be happy for a visitor. Plus I want to tell him the news.

Sitting across from him at dinner in my mom's spot, I pour him a glass of wine, slide his plate toward me, cut his chicken for him, slide the plate back.

"Where is your wine glass?" he asks. And I tell him, "I'm not drinking right now. Because I'm going to have a baby."

The crevices of his face twist into a smile. He doesn't say any of the usual things: "Congratulations" or "How are you feeling?" or "When is the due date?" He tells me he is pleased, and he asks if I've told Mom. "Yes, she knows."

He pauses for a moment and smiles, gives a little chuckle. Then he starts telling me about his acid reflux, and the subject is closed.

The next morning I find him at the table in his bathrobe, eating the breakfast his caretaker has prepared for him. His usual: a slice of walnut levain bread and half a can of sardines, a bottle of warm beer. I fix myself a bowl of muesli and sit across from him. He tells me he didn't sleep well last night. "I was thinking about things that kept me awake. Including ... what you told me."

I smile. "You mean about the baby?"

He nods, his face serious.

"You were thinking about it in a good way, right?"

"Oh, yes," he says. Then he starts talking about what a wonderful thing it is when children are "wanted." He recalls a time in the early nineties when all the newspapers were reporting the same remarkable finding: a sharp and consistent drop in crime rates around the country. "And this was correlated with, you know, the abortion decision in the Supreme Court, some twenty years earlier."

"Roe v. Wade," I say.

"Yes." And he makes one of his faces, this kind of satisfied pout—eyebrows up, corners of the mouth turned down—meaning he has considered the evidence and finds it persuasive. *You can't argue with that.*

Then he asks me if I've ever read the novel *Effi Briest.* I tell him I think so. "I remember you told both

127

of us to read it when we were in high school. I think I did, but I'm not sure. I don't remember it."

He recalls the plot for me: Effi Briest is a well-to-do young woman, pregnant with her first child, when she hires a young maid, Rosvilda, to work in her home. Rosvilda has a young child of her own. She turns out to be a devoted servant. The two women become friends; Rosvilda sticks by Effie's side after Effie's husband throws her out of the house for some past infidelity. Gradually Effie gets to know her maid's life story: when Rosvilda became pregnant as a girl, out of wedlock—here my dad starts to cry, searching for his hanky and blowing his nose before continuing—"Her father, who was a blacksmith, when he heard about her state, he came after her with a hot iron. He attacked her." He makes a jabbing motion in the air with his right hand, to demonstrate. "Which, of course, is frightening to any young woman, but especially to a pregnant woman, with a baby inside of her." He shakes his head and blows his nose again, and I have this distinct thought: *He really is capable of empathy, of putting himself in someone else's shoes, even someone quite different from himself, and feeling deep compassion for them. And yet he seems so incapable of that sometimes with his own wife and daughters.*

"So, anyway," he concludes, "it is a good thing when children are wanted and everyone is happy about it." He smiles mischievously. "I, at least, will not be coming after you with a hot iron."

We both laugh over that. "Well," I say, "I guess that's a good start."

On my drive home in the late afternoon, Simon and Garfunkel's "The Boxer" comes on the radio. It's a song I used to listen to over and over in college, always wondering about the meaning, loving and hating the sadness of it. Today it seems as if the song were written about my dad: all the physical blows his body has taken over the past twelve years, and how he keeps going on, dogged, insistent, stupidly stubborn. I can see this image of him in a ring, bloodied and beaten, almost bent double in his weakness; he keeps getting knocked down, over and over, and still he struggles back to his feet, hungry, ready to take the next blow.

And in the same moment I am thinking about being a mother, and the love parents have for their children. I press my hand to my belly below my seatbelt, and I feel the weight and the hope of this wanted child.

SIXTEEN WEEKS

I ALWAYS GIVE MY patients the same advice at their first prenatal visit: "The first trimester is when the risk of miscarriage is the highest. Of course you'll want to share your news with family and friends. But remember that it's still early. For now, I suggest that you only talk about the pregnancy with people you could imagine talking about a miscarriage with."

The very young ones sometimes look at me sheepishly and admit they've already posted it on Facebook. The older women, the ones who have miscarried before or know someone who has, are more cautious. They nod gravely. "Of course," they say. "Of course."

In the second trimester, after checking for the fetal heartbeat, I tell them that things are looking good, and I encourage them to share their happy news if they haven't already.

For most women (and for me, it turns out), the second trimester is a glorious time. I'm nowhere close to visibly pregnant, but I can press my hand below my navel and feel the firm top of my uterus beginning to rise up out of my pelvis. The fetus inside me is no larger than a baseball. Even though I can't yet feel it move, on the ultrasound I can see it kicking and somersaulting. It will be another month or maybe longer before those kicks are strong enough to reverberate through the thick muscular uterine wall, creating the thuds and flutters that will be the constant reassurance of the growing life inside me.

The truth is that a miscarriage can happen at any time. There are no promises, ever.

At sixteen weeks, a fetus is still a primitive nervous system, incapable of feeling pain or surviving for more than a few seconds outside the womb. But visually, it is a fully formed human being, with ten fingers and ten toes, delicate facial bones and lips puckered in a permanent, curious kiss.

Last week during a routine D&E procedure, a sixteen-week fetus came out intact. I dropped it in the metal dish and I saw it move, or I thought I saw it move.

It was all I could do not to vomit, to run from the room crying.

It's been a long, wet spring. Recently the cat has been bringing salamanders into the house. One morning I rise early, walk into the kitchen, and find one of these awful creatures, gummy and translucent with its enormous black eyeballs, writhing and twitching on the floor. I can't stand to look at it. I yell, unfairly, at the cat, and squeeze my eyes shut while I wait for Mo to come take the thing away.

In September, just a few months into my intern year, one of our co-residents announced that she was pregnant. She had just entered her second trimester, about sixteen weeks. She was due in February.

Kaitlyn and I weren't close, but we spent a lot of time together because we happened to share the same hospital schedule: on any given month, we were usually the two interns on a particular service together. She was slender and pretty in an understated way, with pale blond hair, straight-across bangs, and a smile as wide as a slice of watermelon. She was from Chicago, and she had that open, Midwestern kindness about her, but without any old-fashioned propriety. She wasn't the type of person who hid her problems, trying to be perfect. Nevertheless, she had a natural perfection about her, like a beautiful woman who can go without makeup. Early in our first year, she had already distinguished herself as one of the most capable interns. Working alongside her at neighboring computers or passing her in the hallway, I would often ask her how to do something—set up home nursing appointments for a patient, or which blood pressure drug to use in someone with lupus. She knew her medicine better than I did, better than most of us, and she'd already figured out how to do most things in the hospital. She always stopped to help me as though she had all the time in the world, never showing a trace of impatience. Maybe she simply didn't find the work as stressful as I did. Still, I couldn't imagine how anyone, even Kaitlyn, would choose to have a baby while doing this job.

One afternoon that fall, we were walking down to the cafeteria together, rushing to get there before the lunch service closed—after which we would be stuck with the limp, cellophane-wrapped sandwiches and apples they left out for desperate residents. She was barely showing yet, but as we crossed the hospital courtyard splashed with yellow gingko leaves, I noticed she was already breathing more heavily, with those deep, determined breaths of a healthy pregnant woman.

We loaded our plates and sat down at a picnic table in the courtyard. Between bites of pasta salad and soggy squash, I asked her how long she'd been trying to get pregnant.

"Oh, I wasn't trying," she said with an ironic laugh. "No no no. I was on birth control. But I was working nights, and then I was moving across the country to start residency, and my schedule got all thrown off. I was late taking a pill. One pill." She rolled her eyes deep into her forehead. "Are you kidding me, Chris? This couldn't have happened at a worse time." She told me she was in the process of divorcing her husband. "The day I kicked him out of the house and called a lawyer," she said, "was the day I realized my period was a week late."

The most obvious question was already on my lips, but I knew better than to ask it: *Why didn't you just get an abortion?* I guessed the answer was simple: she'd rather have the baby.

She had made a choice I could not imagine myself making, not in a thousand years. I can see now how superior I felt: I held my IUD like a prize inside of me. I had thought this was what made us—women like me and Kaitlyn—different from our patients: I believed we had somehow earned happiness by making smart choices, the right choices, rather than being pushed and pulled at the mercy of fate and circumstance. Prevention was just another thing we were good at. Now in the midst of a divorce and a grueling residency, with her family halfway across the country, Kaitlyn was going to continue a pregnancy she hadn't planned on, and have a baby she hadn't wanted in the first place.

But it was obvious, even to me, that she wanted it now. It radiated off of her like her warmth and intelligence. It was just another thing she wore with perfect ease: motherhood.

I felt it like a great distance, a wide open plain between us.

In the meantime I had my own pregnant patients to care for.

Many of the young patients in our clinic were immigrants and refugees. One day shortly after Kaitlyn's announcement, a Sudanese woman came to see me, pregnant with her second child. Her pelvic exam wasn't normal. The skin was too tight; the vaginal opening too small and round. Instead of the center of an unfolding flower or a pea pod, her vagina looked like the lens of a camera or the barrel of a gun. Something man-made, designed for a man's use.

I was even more puzzled because she'd had a baby before—a boy, now four years old, born vaginally. How, I wondered, could a baby have passed through this strange, small aperture?

I didn't ask. I didn't even mention the exam. To my surprise, I was able to pass a speculum (the "duck bill" instrument that separates the vaginal walls) inside and see her cervix, which was round and plump and snugly closed. By the measurements of her ultrasound, she was twelve weeks pregnant. I figured I had plenty of time before I had to address the issue. I pulled the drape over her lap, helped her up, and told her I would step out while she dressed. Then I returned to discuss the details of the pregnancy.

Her husband was there with her, holding their little boy, quiet and saucer-eyed, in his arms. The husband was quiet, too, saying little except when she or I asked him to translate a word. (His English was perfect; hers was not.) They had been resettled here just over a year ago, they told me. He had recently found regular work, and they were ready for a second child. He was tall and thin but broad-chested, in a long cotton robe and skull cap. His wiry black beard hung to the base of his throat; I noticed a few strands of gray in it. But his skin was youthful, smooth and brown. His eyes were boyish and kind. Her chart said she was twenty-four; I guessed he wasn't much older.

At the end of the visit, I congratulated them, touched her shoulder, then held my hand out to him. He took a step back, folding his hands together at his chest. "I'm sorry, Doctor. I do not touch any woman besides my wife. It is our religious custom."

Like a reflex, my intellectual, feminist brain reeled at the rebuke. But in the same instant, my heart softened toward him. Even in the act of rejecting a handshake, he managed to convey a sense of respect and humility. His hands, fingers interlaced at his heart, conveyed a gesture of prayer or supplication. A humble request.

I lifted my hand from its angle at my side, holding my palm up to him in what I hoped was a gesture of acceptance. "Of course," I said. "It's no problem. Well, congratulations to you."

She came alone, by bus, to her next appointment. I was glad. I had come prepared to discuss what I had seen the last time, and I felt emboldened by the absence of anyone else, any man, in the room.

After checking the fetal heartbeat and reviewing her labs and weight, I sat with her and asked a simple but direct question: "When you were in the Sudan, was your vagina cut and sewn together again?"

For a second she gave me a blank look, and I feared I was mistaken. What if she said no? What if this was simply how her body looked? Was that even possible? Maybe. I had only read about female circumcision. I had never seen it before. I was just an intern. What did I know?

But then she said, in the most matter-of-fact voice, "Yes." As though I had asked her whether she had had breakfast that morning. "Before the baby, when I was fourteen years old. And again, after my son was born. They sewed me back up."

I nodded. "Yes. I thought so."

There was a brief silence. I considered asking her who did this to her. A midwife? Village elders? Her own mother? But I resisted the temptation of my own curiosity. It made no difference to our work together.

She broke the silence. "Actually, I want to ask you," she said. "Will it be a problem? For the baby to come out?"

I had wondered the same thing, and I was prepared to answer her. After our last appointment, I'd sought out an attending physician who had worked in the Sudan with Doctors Without Borders, and I'd asked her what she knew about female circumcision. What had to be done in childbirth to get the baby out?

"Ninety-eight percent of the time, nothing," she said. "In the vast majority of these women, it's just the labia that have been sewn together, very superficially. The introitus looks small, but behind it, the vaginal canal is plenty big enough for the baby's head to pass. Once it reaches the perineum, everything just stretches and expands like in any other woman. I've never even had to cut an episiotomy in any of these patients— although you always have that option if you need it.

Tell her there's nothing to worry about. She can have her baby just like anyone else."

So, like a good resident, in a voice as confident as if I had answered this question a thousand times, I told her exactly what I had learned from my attending a few weeks earlier. "It won't be a problem," I concluded after a brief explanation. "The baby will come out."

She nodded. "It came out the first time. But I was young then, and I don't remember much. The nurse didn't tell me what she was doing—it just happened." Then she looked at me. "Will you be there with me? When the baby comes?"

"Of course," I said. "I will be there."

But instead of looking relieved, she still seemed anxious. "And after?" she asked.

"After?"

"After the baby is out. Will you leave me as I am, or will you sew me back together?"

This was a question I had not considered. I paused for a moment, then asked, "What would you like me to do?"

She looked down. "I don't know. I don't know if we will have more children after this one. But I have always been this way, for as long as I remember."

"And sex with your husband?" I asked. "Is it …"

"Fine," she said. "Not painful. It is good."

"And does he ..." I hesitated. "Does he have an opinion?"

She shook her head. "No. He told me he doesn't mind. He says it is my body. He just wants me and the baby to be healthy."

I thought of this man, tall and young and serious, who would not shake my hand. I thought, *He knows more about what it means to be a man than most of the men in our supposedly enlightened West.*

"I agree with him," I said, with a firm nod. "Anyway, you don't have to decide now. I will do whatever you ask me to do. Every woman has a right to have her vagina look and work after childbirth the way it did before. So if you ask me to sew it up, I will. If you ask me to leave it, I will."

She nodded. "Thank you."

After thinking for a moment, I said, "But listen, I'm not a plastic surgeon." In my mind, I added: *And I'm no believer in your customs, the things that were done to you when you were fourteen.* "I can sew you up right after the delivery, if that's what you want. But not six months later. So try to decide beforehand what you want me to do. Okay?"

She laughed, the look of relief I had hoped for flooding her brown eyes. "I understand," she said.

I saw her every month throughout her pregnancy. Usually her husband managed to take time off work to accompany her. As with most of my prenatal patients, I grew fond of her; we hugged hello and goodbye at every visit. I felt awkward giving her husband just a nod of greeting, but he managed to smooth it over with his poise. I began to feel close to him, too, despite the invisible wall between us.

One afternoon in April, close to her due date, I was called to Labor & Delivery. She had come in dilated and pushing. The perineum was already stretched and thinning into a pale ring of tissue that I knew would allow the head to pass. I placed my gloved fingers on the dark, damp ellipse of skull and held her gaze. "Are you ready for the last push?"

She winced, nodded.

"Yes? Good."

She delivered a healthy baby girl, fists pumping and mouth wide open, wailing in delight at her new world.

The perineum tore about a centimeter posteriorly, but the bleeding stopped on its own, probably stemmed by the matrix of collagen scar embedded in the tissue. She asked me not to sew her together.

I gave a little smile. "Are you planning a third child?"

A look of horror crossed her face. "Oh God," she said. "Not soon." Then the corners of her mouth twitched upward. "Maybe in the future."

I stripped off my gown and gloves and washed up to my elbows in the sink, while her husband performed a short prayer ritual over the baby, singing to her in a language I had never heard and never have since. When I returned to the bedside, the baby was cuddled to her mother's breast, sucking. The husband stood as always, tall and silent, holding their son in his arms. "I'll leave you in peace and come visit you tomorrow," I said to her. "Congratulations." She looked at me for a moment, then gazed back down at her baby.

"Thank you, doctor," her husband said, his eyes wide and damp.

I beamed at him, reached out and clapped him on the shoulder with a firm, congratulatory slap of my palm. Then I drew back, whisking my hand to my mouth. "Oh gosh! I'm sorry! I didn't—I forgot!"

He laughed, his teeth shining. "It is no problem," he said. "It really is no problem. Thank you for everything."

I laced my fingers at the level of my heart, imitating the gesture he had made that first day, and gave a little nod, my own humble request. "It's my pleasure."

The other residents were enamored of the idea of Kaitlyn's coming baby. There was constant talk about it in the resident lounge and elevators, especially among the women. She moved out of the house she'd rented with her husband into an apartment a few blocks from the hospital. One weekend some of the interns helped her decorate the spare room as a nursery. As her due date approached, they set up a post-partum meal delivery schedule; I signed up to bring her lentil soup and salad one night. There was even talk of putting together a babysitting spreadsheet so we could all volunteer to help when Kaitlyn came back to work, but I drew the line there. I didn't see why, with my scarce free time, I should sign up to take care of another resident's baby.

Despite her readiness, her proud, gravid abdomen, and her dogged work ethic (she still seemed to get her work done faster and better than I did, even in her eighth month of pregnancy), I thought Kaitlyn didn't quite know what she was getting herself into. I still believed she had made the wrong choice.

I didn't attend the baby shower, even though I had the day off. I don't remember what I did instead. Probably I was writing or swimming laps—the things I always did, the routines I clung to because they gave me some illusion of control.

I happened to be on call the night Kaitlyn had her baby.

The hospital was packed, busy, chaotic. It was a long, cold night in the middle of a wet winter; homeless and elderly patients kept flooding into the ER. I was working downstairs admitting patients to the hospital, but I saw on the computer admission log that Kaitlyn was upstairs in Labor & Delivery. I didn't have much time to think about it. I remember vaguely hoping that things went smoothly for her. Then I got back to my work.

In the early morning, I was in the ER examining a drunk and obnoxious man with alcoholic cirrhosis, my last admission of the night, when the Code Blue signal came over the P.A. system. I excused myself and broke into a jog, mindlessly following the voice to the specified unit of the hospital. The three beeps kept repeating and the lights kept flashing, and I pounded up the stairs as I always did. As my footsteps echoed against the concrete steps and walls, they were joined by the footsteps of my co-interns, who were just arriving in this dim hour of morning to begin their long day of work, all of us merging into the thundering chorus of another morning at the hospital. I was secretly glad for the interruption, hoping the Code Blue would delay the admission just long enough that a daytime resident would offer to take it off my hands.

It did not occur to me until we rounded the corner onto the unit where we were headed: Labor & Delivery. Then I realized that none of them knew it either. They had all just arrived; they didn't know who had been laboring here all night. "Oh shit," I said under my breath. "Kaitlyn." I felt the weight and the dread of it crash on me like a wave.

At the door to the operating room, a nurse blocked our entrance. "It's okay," she kept saying. "It's okay. It's not her. It's the baby." And then we all knew.

We waited together. We could see through the small window of the operating room door. The pediatricians were hovering around the warmer, hiding the baby from view. Kaitlyn was on the operating table; they were sewing her back up. I have never felt as close to my co-residents as I felt during those few minutes, because the stakes were the same for all of us. We were all crashing under that wave together, clutching one another, even though I don't remember touching a single person, just watching through that clear rectangle.

I am no pediatrician. I was barely even a doctor, then. But when I saw them wheel that baby out of the operating room—its head swollen like a grotesque balloon, blue veins visible under its taut, translucent skin—I knew what was going to happen. I knew it didn't matter what choices Kaitlyn had made or what choices she would make in the future. Her choices meant nothing anymore.

It is impossible to write about a baby who dies on the day it's born. It's like trying to take in all the air in the atmosphere in one breath. It is the shortest story and the longest story in the whole world.

I have written about that night more times than I can remember. No matter how many words or how few, it is never enough.

So why am I trying again now?

Because now I am sixteen weeks pregnant. I've made it through the first trimester and all the terror that came with it, my heart in my throat every time I pulled down my underwear, fearing I would see blood.

But now that I've made it beyond those tenuous early weeks, I am somewhere even more terrifying: back in that ocean where I was that night, the dread of a wave about to crash and knowing the breath will be knocked out of me when it does.

Now I see that the reason Kaitlyn's choice bothered me was because I took it as a betrayal, a crossing to the other side. Not just that she was leaving the life of a young, independent woman to become a mother, although there was that. But more important, it was the crossing from a place of control to a place of vulnerability, putting her life in the hands of fate and circumstance. I think I understood, on some level, that the moment Kaitlyn chose to keep her pregnancy was the moment she gave up all other choices. She could continue to be the woman she was, but from that moment on she would always be living her life for her child. And that is exactly what happened. She chose motherhood, and her baby died. And then she still had to live with that choice. I know Kaitlyn is still living for that child, will live for it and with it forever.

Now I have made that choice, too.

In abortion care, a sixteen-week fetus is not a child. But this life inside of me—it is a child. It is my child. I am already radiating with that certainty, just like Kaitlyn did that afternoon in the courtyard, while I sat there judging her.

Although I can't feel it moving, most of the time I am able to reassure myself that it's there, it's alive. But some evenings after the patients have gone home, I start to worry so much I can't stand it. Then I close the door to my office, press the Doppler probe to my abdomen and find the heartbeat, fast and steady, a horse beating a gallop across an open plain.

A few months later, I was back working on Labor & Delivery, where Kaitlyn and her dead baby were always with me, like the blood on my shoes and the tangy smell of birth on my forearms. Instead of sadness, I felt a deep chill, a nothingness that pervaded every waking and sleeping minute, both in and out of the hospital.

In the hours when I wasn't working, I drifted in and out of our house in a daze. One night I arrived home after finishing a shift at 8 p.m. Mo was at the gym. I always went to bed early on nights like these, anxious to get a good night's sleep. As I walked into the empty house, I imagined how I would spend the short time alone: a cup of tea, an apple cut in thin slices, an hour of writing in bed. First I had to finish some notes on the last of the day's deliveries. I sat down at the kitchen table with my laptop and tried to sign into the hospital network. The screen blinked an error message. I tried again. *Error.*

Forty-five minutes later I was still sitting there. Mo came home. I heard his gym bag land on the floor.

"Hi," I said without looking up from the screen, which was prompting me for the third time to create a new password.

He came straight over to me and put a hand on my head. I raised my cheek to let him kiss it. "You eat?" he asked.

"Yeah, at the hospital."

He kept standing there next to me. "Can I make you some tea or something?"

"No thanks," I said, still not looking at him. Then I added, "Sorry, I'm just stressed."

He kept his hand on my hair. "Is there anything I can do to un-stress you?"

I almost screamed, almost pushed him away. His gentleness, his kindness, his desire to help—it was horrible. *Don't you get it? Don't you understand? There is nothing you can do. Just leave me alone. Alone. Alone.*

I didn't say anything, just sat there, my hands motionless on the keyboard, until he left. When he was sitting on the couch doing his own work, I closed my computer and stood up. I could finish the stupid notes tomorrow.

I knew what was the right thing to do. I simply needed to say, "I changed my mind. Would you mind making me a cup of tea and cutting up an apple and bringing it to me in bed?" Ridiculous as it may have been, he would have been thrilled to do this for me. I could have crawled under the covers and he would have brought me my special mug and the apple slices on a little plate, and he would have loved doing it, loved me for letting him do it.

Instead I walked into the kitchen and turned on the faucet. The water splashed, loud and cruel, in the bottom of the tea kettle. I knew he could hear it, and I knew I had done the most rotten thing, as awful as if I had spat in his face.

In the middle of the following night, we took a patient back to the OR for a C-section after she'd been pushing for three hours with no progress.

I stood in the primary surgeon spot with Dr. K assisting me. I got into the uterus easily, but when I reached in to deliver the head, all I could feel was a shoulder. The fetal head was well below the incision, already deep in the woman's pelvis after three hours of pushing. I couldn't even find it with my fingertips. Dr. K reached in and he couldn't grab it either. He told a nurse to crawl under the drape and push the head up from below. It probably took less than a minute, but it felt much longer.

Finally Dr. K was able to grab something. With some grunting and straining, his arm up to the elbow in the woman's body, he pulled the baby out and passed it to the waiting pediatrician. It looked tiny and blue and floppy, but many babies look that way in the first moments after a C-section. We turned back to the surgical field. I started suturing the uterus. In the background, I began to hear the voice of the pediatrician chanting softly,

"One and two and three and breathe. One and two and three and breathe." CPR.

Dr. K told me to switch spots with him; he took over sewing the uterus. I couldn't see that it was a particularly difficult closure, but I figured there must be something I was missing. I stepped aside, held the bladder blade, and kept listening to the voices of the nursery team over my shoulder: "One and two and three and breathe."

Dr. K kept looking up from the field to the back corner of the room. I realized he was looking at the baby, checking to see if they were still doing chest compressions. Dr. K was one of the most risk-conscious physicians in the hospital. He was always talking to us about how to practice so as not to get sued. I wondered if he was thinking about the baby or about the progression of the woman's labor, whether he should have taken her back to the operating room sooner, whether he could be accused of having done something wrong. Whatever it was, it was clear that he wanted to be in control of something in that moment, tying tiny knots—more perfect knots than I would've tied—instead of just standing there watching, wondering if the baby was going to die.

I also noticed the baby's father. He'd been standing up and looking over the drape the entire time, watching us as we operated. Most dads stayed crouched behind the sheet beside the mother, whispering to her and calming her down. But he had watched with interest as we made the first skin incision, dissected through the layers of fascia, separated the abdominal muscles. I'd stopped paying attention, but I assumed he had been watching during those long, chaotic moments as we struggled to pull out the baby.

As I stood there watching Dr. K suture and listening to the voices chanting and reciting the events of the baby's resuscitation—"Still no heartbeat ... We're at two minutes ... One and two and three and breathe" —I became aware of the father again, watching silently, wide-eyed, over the top of the drape.

Soon the counting stopped, and I heard them calling out the baby's heart rate and discussing other technicalities of the resuscitation. A minute later the baby was whisked out of the OR on the warmer, alarms beeping and cords flying and trailing behind. I remembered Kaitlyn's baby. "Henneberg," Dr. K said, nodding to me. "Suture scissors, please." I handed them to him.

He continued tying knots and blotting and burning tiny blood vessels with the cauterizing blade. I heard people saying the baby was doing better in the nursery. "He's breathing on his own." "Apgars were one, five, seven." (A way of saying his neonatal well-being scores were quickly improving.) Someone came to take the father to the nursery, so his stricken face was no longer hovering over us. I heard the anesthesiologist offer the mother "something to help you relax," and her weak voice accepting. Soon she was snoring.

After that Dr. K let me finish the rest of the closure. I forgot about the baby, just focused on tying knots in straight little rows. Dr. K gave me some pointers on my technique. We cracked a few jokes about other things, mundane things. Then that satisfying act of blotting away the last bits of dried blood with clean white towels, the sticky removal of the drape, the woman's abdomen wrinkled and soft where it had been stretched taut just thirty minutes ago. We threw our bloody gloves in the trash.

Afterward, I went to the nursery to see the baby. The father stood there staring down at him, his arms crossed over his chest. "I just hate to see him like this," he said to me, or maybe to no one in particular.

I shrugged. I thought the baby looked pink and strong despite all the lines and the little mask strapped to his face. "Most of that stuff is just monitoring him at this point," I said. "He's doing pretty much everything on his own now. Soon they'll be able to take all that stuff off."

The rest of the night was quiet. I wrote the operative note and sent it to Dr. K to review, then fell onto the couch in the call room and slept for four hours, the longest I'd ever slept on Labor & Delivery. When I emerged into the hallway in the early morning, I heard the nurses talking about the case earlier in the night. "Ambulance just left. They took the baby to Children's Hospital for brain cooling."

"Oh, shit," another nurse said. "That's bad. That kid's probably gonna have cerebral palsy."

I felt as though they were talking about something that had nothing to do with me, something I knew nothing about. I'd just slept for four hours and woken up feeling amazing. Somehow I'd thought it had been a normal night, a good night. Why was I only realizing, gradually and stupidly, that something terrible had happened? Brain cooling was a process meant to minimize long-term damage from hypoxic brain injury. If the nurses were right—and even if they weren't—a happily anticipated event for this young couple had turned out to be an event of trauma and loss, nothing like what they'd expected, exactly what they'd never let themselves imagine.

What had I been thinking about while I was lying on the couch, drifting into my crooked half-sleep? I had been thinking about myself, as usual. I had been trying, once again, to figure out if I was truly unhappy. *No*, I thought. *I'm too busy to be unhappy. I'm just tired and numb.*

The next day, a Sunday, I slept until three and woke to a bright, windy afternoon. I walked down to the waterfront, but instead of making my usual loop on the quiet dirt path, I cut through the park. It was full of people of all ages. I passed the bocce courts, where a tournament of sorts seemed to be going on, and the playground, which was crawling with toddlers and their mothers. At the baseball diamonds, three different games were in play—two of teenage boys in team uniforms, one of men in shorts and T-shirts. I leaned against the fence like a kid, the railing tucked under my armpits, to watch one of the boys' games. Things seemed to move more quickly than in baseball games on TV, because the ball was dropped every now and then and someone needed to chase it. The runners advanced along the bases. The parents in the bleachers yelled, "Go! Go!" and the boys yelped and shouted at one another.

I cut across an empty soccer field and headed back toward the water—past the yacht club and the Marina Market Bait & Tackle Shop, where a sign in the window read:

CHIPS
COLD BEER
LIVE BAIT
HOT COFFEE

At the dock, a lone fishing boat was tied up. The water lapped at the concrete, and the little boat rocked gently, like a lullaby. My eyes and legs suddenly felt tired. I walked out onto the wooden dock, just next to where the boat bobbed on the water, and sat down. I tucked my hands under my legs and hummed to myself.

Sittin' here restin' my bones,
And this loneliness won't leave me alone.

There was a loneliness there with me that was difficult to place. It had something to do with working all night and sleeping through most of this sunny day— and then being in such close proximity to these people and their communal weekend activities: ball games, picnics, moms pushing their kids on the swing set and chatting over their shoulders.

I thought about the night I'd spent on Labor & Delivery and what strange and isolating work it was: gazing at the computerized strips on the wall, occasionally entering one of the patient's rooms to slip my fingers around the edge of her cervix or break a bag of water. Sleeping on the couch in the resident lounge with my pager glowing on the table next to me. The babies I'd delivered, including the one who was at this minute lying on a tiny bed in Children's Hospital, where they were freezing his oxygen-starved brain cells, chilling him like a piece of fruit picked too soon from the tree.

As I sat on the dock in my circadian stupor, hypnotized by the motion of the water, I couldn't have felt further away from the people around me in the park, their lives and activities and joys and worries.

A car engine rumbled in the parking lot behind me, coming closer. I turned and saw an old van with a boat trailer rigged up behind it reversing alongside the dock, the trailer aimed toward the boat in the water. When the trailer was mostly submerged, almost touching the boat, a man climbed out the driver's side and walked onto the dock. He had a thick white beard and wore black rubber boots, jeans with suspenders, a backwards ratty baseball cap and sunglasses pushed up on his forehead. He was tall and his arms were brown and strong. Although he passed right by me, he didn't say a word or even turn his head. A cigarette was caught in his lips, and it remained there as he untied the boat from the dock and, gripping the ropes in both hands, guided the boat expertly onto the trailer. As he worked, I turned and peered inside the passenger window of the van. On the dashboard: a pack of cigarettes, a water bottle, an empty tin can. I imagined the can served as a receptacle of some kind, maybe for chewing tobacco or cigarette butts.

Now the boat was secured to the trailer. The man walked by me again without saying a word, cigarette in his lips. He climbed into the van and drove away, the little boat rattling behind on the trailer. I wondered where he was going now, and what it would have been like to spend this sunny day out on the water in that boat, with piles of fish in old paint buckets, a pack of cigarettes in a Ziplock bag.

Memorial Day weekend. On our one-year wedding anniversary, Mo and I flew to Philadelphia. Margot, one of my best friends from college, was getting married. Mo didn't know Margot well. She and I had been closest during our senior year, after Mo graduated, when I had drifted away from him and told him I wanted us to see other people. I think he distrusted Margot because of that. It was true that she had urged me to enjoy being single in our last year of college, and I had—although I'd missed Mo. I worried that he still felt the sting of that old rejection whenever I pulled away from him in bed, or shrugged off his touch.

Sitting there on the plane next to my husband, I remembered something my dad once said to me: "You have to watch out, Chrissy, because you are the kind of strong-willed woman who will push around a nice guy like Mo. He won't stand up to you, because he's too nice. But in the end, you will make him miserable."

I had wanted to sleep on the flight, but instead Mo dozed off beside me and I sat there thinking about things I hadn't thought about in months, the events in the weeks leading up to our wedding. In the roaring silence of the engines, I closed my eyes, but the memories slipped under my eyelids, returning to me. The TV screen flickering on Mo's eyes at the Marriott, my hand reaching for his under the sheets. Mo's voice on the phone on a Sunday morning, two weeks before the wedding: "It's about Neil." The carpet under my knees as I said, "Oh God, Oh God, Oh God." And something I had not witnessed but could see as clearly as any memory: Mo's mom walking into a dark living room and finding her nephew's body hanging from the chandelier hook, his feet turning in a slow circle.

These things struck me almost as new discoveries, as though I were just learning that they had actually happened, or that we had lived through them.

I thought of a study I'd read in medical school about patients who survive hospitalization in the ICU and return home, only to suffer from PTSD-like symptoms: paralyzing anxiety, irritability, nightmares in which they relived the agonizing delirium of critical illness and sedation. Alive but not alive, breathing through a tube, vessels clamped by chemicals, heart flogged by an adrenaline whip.

I had heard that Kaitlyn was undergoing a specific type of PTSD therapy, in which she was made to relive over and over again the events that had happened the night of her baby's birth, to feel the things she had felt as they were unfolding. It had happened only three months ago. Three months ago her baby had died. How could she be expected to know what she was thinking or feeling at the time? Hadn't she barely even begun to realize that it had happened, that it was real? That she'd lived through it?

I woke up late the morning of Margot's wedding and groggily presented myself for my bridal party duties.

At the reception dinner, I sat looking around the hall as more of our college friends moved onto the dance floor.

"Want to dance?" Mo asked.

"I don't feel like it. I don't mind if you do," I said.

He shook his head. "No, I'll stick with you."

I sat there watching Laura Langley and Stacey Moore, two other women from our college class who were close to Margot, though I didn't know them well. They'd both had children in the past few years, but they were gorgeous and thin, dancing in short dresses with blond hair down their backs, their legs perfectly tanned. At the rehearsal dinner the night before, they'd both mentioned that they worked "part time"— which I suspected meant hardly at all. I felt strangely jealous of them for having something I wanted, and simultaneously proud of myself for choosing something different. (Maybe there was a German word for this.) Even though I had bags under my eyes and my legs were pale and I hadn't exercised in weeks, I felt proud of my hard work over the past several years, of having acquired a body of knowledge and a set of skills that allowed me to do meaningful work, even if it wasn't work I liked doing. This was what I would have to give up if I left medicine, I thought—not just the work, but my pride in the work.

I knew a risk of leaving medicine was that I would turn my focus onto other matters of pride, such as money and beauty. Sitting there next to Mo, saying nothing, I felt better than I'd expected to feel that evening. I felt good about being just another pleasant, pale-legged lady at a wedding, licking cake icing off her fork, loving her husband, and looking forward to going to bed early, taking a Benadryl and sleeping like the dead.

At the airport the next day, waiting for our flight to board, Mo told me he was unhappy in our marriage. He didn't raise it as an urgent issue. He said it almost casually, his feet propped on his rollaway bag. *I would like to feel more loved by you.*

I couldn't get him to give me more specifics. He mentioned wishing we had spent more time together on this trip. He mentioned sex. At one point he said, "We had something great in the past, and I know we can have something great again in the future."

"So, you feel like our marriage isn't great now?" I asked.

"Not really," he said.

On the flight home, we sat next to each other in silence. Once again he fell asleep, and I sat there awake, staring at nothing, turning it all over in my mind. The thing that saddened and confused me the most was that I did think our marriage was great and strong. But apparently I was alone in that feeling. And even worse, he was alone. All this time he had been living alone in an unhappy marriage.

After all my doubt and ambivalence, I felt finally, definitely sure of what the problem was: it was residency. It wasn't just the hours and the exhaustion. My intern year—the hardest year—was nearly behind me. I knew I could finish two more years. I was even starting to think I could be a good doctor. But I could not do it and keep alive the other parts of myself and my life that were most important to me: my marriage, my family, my writing.

The worst thing was this: If all I had to do was get through these next two years and then be a doctor and a writer, that would be fine. Even to be a doctor, a writer, and a wife seemed feasible.

But I had yet to face the biggest, most demanding, most important role of all: to be a mother.

I thought of Laura Langley and Stacey Moore and the babies they bounced on their movie star hips. I thought of Denise Winters and the way her mother slept curled in the armchair at her bedside. I remembered Dr. W's admonition: *When you are a mother yourself, then you'll understand.*

And now Mo was telling me he didn't feel loved by me. All along I had been saying, "I'm losing my words! I'm losing my words!" And what I should have been saying was, "I'm losing my husband! I'm losing my husband!"

The following weekend, we went out to a cheesy Italian restaurant to celebrate our anniversary: a bottle of wine, ravioli, tiramisu. Mo asked me what I was thinking about. I told him I was thinking about Neil.

"What about Neil?"

I gulped my wine, gathering courage. "About the end of his life. That it was a sad ending, but that it was also a very hard life—kind of a sad life. A life of difficulty and pain. Maybe the fact of that difficulty makes the end of his life, I don't know … a little less sad."

He nodded. "Yeah." He seemed to know what I meant, or in any case he didn't seem offended by it.

I went on. "Part of what felt so awful about it, to me, was the contrast: that our wedding was this thing that represented everything we wanted and hoped for, and Neil's death was the opposite." I looked at him. "I don't know what makes a good life, a happy life. You know? I've always felt like it's at least partly about the choices we make. Choosing your career. Choosing your partner. Choosing to be happy or sad, choosing to have regrets or to just keep looking to the future.

But sometimes it seems like it's not about choices at all, you know? It's about things you can't choose, things you can't control. At least that's how it seemed to be for Neil."

He said, "How do you think it is for us?"

I shook my head. "I don't know. I guess I don't know what else to do except to keep trying to make the right choices. It seems like all I can do."

He said, "I guess that's all I can do, too."

A few days later I knocked on the office door of Dr. Brennan, my residency program director, resolved to tell her my decision.

There was nothing warm or nurturing about our talk. She didn't offer me a cup of tea or a seat on a couch. We sat at a small round table where I'd sat a few times before for resident committee meetings. I told her I was unhappy, and that my unhappiness was threatening my marriage. "It's not the schedule, it's not the hours, it's not anything that I can adjust and make better. I'm not happy doing this."

She didn't try to convince me of anything. She didn't ask whether I was certain that leaving residency would make me happier.

Instead she began by telling me that the contract I'd signed to complete my second year of residency was binding and "difficult to break." Then she told me about her residency.

"When I was a resident, I had a different problem. I loved the work. I loved being in the hospital. I was here all the time, hardly sleeping, hardly doing anything else. I couldn't see what a toll it was taking on me. Eventually my program director called me to his office and 'asked' me to take six weeks off. But it wasn't a request, you know what I mean? I wasn't allowed to say no."

It didn't sound like such a terrible problem to me. I would have loved six weeks off. But I also understood what she was saying, how hard that must have been, the questions it must have raised for her: *Can I really do this? Do I really want to do this? Do other people think I'm capable of doing this?*

Then she told me about the years after she finished residency, when she had her children. She told me that when she returned from maternity leave after having each of her babies, she worked only two half-days a week for several months. Gradually she increased up to three full days a week, which she continued for nine years. "My kids are ten and twelve, now. I only came back to work full time two years ago." This surprised me. I knew Dr. Brennan had been the residency director for only two years. I thought of her as a good doctor and a good teacher. Other people in the hospital— important people—must have seen her that way, too, because they chose her for this job.

After talking about herself for a while (which was a relief—not to be asked to talk about myself the whole time), she asked me what I wanted to do. I told her I still thought the best thing would be to leave. "But I know that might be a short-sighted view," I said. "Mainly because I don't know … I don't know what I would do right now if I left."

"If I remember your residency application," she said, "you're a writer, aren't you?"

I gave a little laugh, looked down at the table. "I'm not sure I could call myself a writer anymore. I certainly haven't been writing much over the past few years. I might waitress for a little while. I used to really like that."

I thought I saw her purse her lips slightly. She told me to take a week off to think about it. "I'm not telling you to take time off," she said. "I'm offering it."

"I'll take it," I said.

I spent that evening and much of the following week at the waterfront, asking the same questions of myself, the hills, the waves at my feet, and always getting the same answer. *I know I will hear what I've heard before.* But I never went back to Dr. Brennan's office.

Instead, the following week I returned to the hospital, still telling myself that I hadn't decided anything, but that I would keep going in the meantime. It was, in a sense, the path of least resistance. I didn't have to explain it or defend it to anyone. I just had to be a better wife to Mo. I would eventually finish residency, and everyone would be proud of me. Instead of seeing regret or weakness, they would see only pride and triumph and a happy ending: a doctor.

Mostly I wrote about the women, the mothers.

But there was one man. Looking back now, I can see how important he was, what a deep impression he made on me. He came into my bed at night, wrapped his arms around me and breathed in my ear. Why did I go to that autopsy? It was a mistake, I thought afterward. It would stay with me my whole life. And now I see that it was necessary. It is one thing to look at an embryo in a plastic dish. It is another to see a human body, a person with whom you'd sat talking just a few days before, dead on a table, sliced open. It began with Kaitlyn, but the point of no return was really the death and the autopsy of Mr. Lu: the breakdown of those clear lines, the tidy boundaries between "me" and "them," the living and the dead.

Most residents never saw the hospital morgue, never even knew where it was.

By that point in residency, the start of my second year, I had been paged from every phone on every floor of the hospital. I knew every single five-digit extension: every nurse's station, the ER (an admission), L&D (a delivery), the microbiology lab (blood culture results), and on and on. But when the pathologist's assistant paged me that morning, it was from an extension I didn't recognize. She told me the autopsy would begin at 1 p.m., and she gave me directions to a locked door. "Just knock and I'll let you in," she said. I had to repeat the directions back to her to make sure I hadn't misunderstood which door she meant. "You mean in the courtyard?"

"That's the one," she said.

I finished my notes, ate a few bites of lunch, and hurried down the hospital stairway. Stepping into the bright afternoon, I followed her directions to a cream-colored door in a shady courtyard, a door we all walked by several times a day—doctors, nurses, visitors, family members—because it was next to the cafeteria. As I stood there, I could hear the clang of the plastic trays being loaded into dishwashers and smell the onion rings in a deep fryer. At a picnic table under an umbrella, the same table where I'd sat with Kaitlyn several months earlier, two residents were scarfing down veggie burgers.

I knocked and the door swung open. A pretty woman in a ponytail, clean hospital scrubs and rubber boots greeted me. "Hi! I'm Nicky, Dr. E's assistant. You're Dr. Henneberg?"

"Hi, yeah. Sorry I'm late. Did you guys start already?"

"Nope! Come on in. We're just doing the external inspection."

I stepped inside the door and around a low wall, the kind that would discreetly hide the toilet in a hotel bathroom. Celine Dion was playing from an iPhone on a shelf.

It was a small room, nothing like the vast, industrial-looking places on TV shows and movies, with endless rows of drawers lining the walls. This place—square, windowless, spotless—was no bigger than our bedroom. It smelled of bleach and preservative, something that reminded me of my first term in medical school and the anatomy lab where we picked at dead bodies, mapping the nerves and arteries in our notebooks with colored pencils.

In the center of the room was a low metal table with a drain at the far end. On the table was Mr. Lu, naked, dead.

The last time I'd seen him was two days ago, as I hurried through my Saturday morning rounds, trying to get home in time to go to the pool before it closed. He was sitting in a chair, his hands in his lap.

Mr. Lu! You're looking so much better! Are you feeling better?

Uh-huh, yeah. I feel little better.

Crouching at his feet, pressing my fingers into his doughy ankles. *Don't you think your legs are getting better? Don't you think they're less swollen?*

Don't know. You're the doctor.

Ha! But they're YOUR legs!

Smiling. *Huh-huh. I guess so. I guess a little better.*

I made it to the pool in time to swim a hundred laps, shower, and sit on the deck for a few minutes to listen to the water lapping at the drain. The P.A. system announced, *Attention swimmers. The pool will be closing in fifteen minutes.* But there were no swimmers, just me sitting on the edge of a lounge chair, my eyes closed, my face toward the sun, when my pager trilled its angry alert from the depths of my gym bag. It was Marcus, the resident covering my patients for the remainder of the weekend. "Hey, Chris. I wanted to let you know about Mr. Lu. Something kind of unexpected happened this afternoon."

Dr. E, the pathologist, was a middle-aged Nigerian man with a broad smile and a thick accent and flecks of gray in his black hair. He wore a clean white dress shirt and gray suit pants. His sleeves were rolled up to the elbow, and he wore a blue plastic apron and long blue gloves. An expensive-looking suit jacket hung over the back of a chair in the corner. He was leaning over the body with a clipboard, taking measurements and directing Nicky to take photographs.

After pausing to introduce himself, he asked me, "Is this your first autopsy?"

"Yes."

"Oh!" His eyes grew wide behind his plastic goggles. "Do you want to take a seat?" He pointed to the chair with the jacket draped over the back.

I shook my head. "No, I'm okay. I don't faint."

He turned back to the body—naked, pale, intact—and Nicky snapped another photograph with the digital camera.

I looked down at Mr. Lu. Suddenly I had more time with him than I'd had during the full week he'd been in the hospital. He'd come into the ER for vague abdominal pain—it turned out he was having a slow myocardial infarction.

Mr. Lu wasn't a typical heart attack patient. He didn't drink or do drugs. He was in his early forties; he'd moved here with his family from China as a boy. His father and an uncle had died young of "heart problems." He lived with his mother and sister; they told us he rarely left the house. He'd had some learning disabilities in school, they said. He went to community college for a year, but had never held a regular job.

We'd kept him in the hospital for several days, giving him diuretics to try to get him out of heart failure before we could transfer him to the nearby private hospital, where they performed cardiac stent procedures. There was nothing for me to do but keep track of his fluid status and make sure he didn't have another heart attack. Under the advice of the cardiologists, I ordered diuretics every morning and checked on his swollen legs and his urine output several times a day. Every day I asked him whether he had any chest pain. "No," he said, his voice dull and distant, like a timid knock on a thick door. "No pain. Just tired."

It was a massive Code Blue, the kind where the whole hospital staff gathers outside the door. Chest compressions for an hour, the beep and burst of the defibrillator, ampules of epinephrine underfoot, doctors and nurses shouting over one another. Marcus wasn't the only resident who told me about it; it seemed like they'd all been there. One told me, "He was saying, 'I can't breathe! I can't breathe!' And then all of a sudden he turned blue, and he was clutching his throat. It was like a movie. It was like, you know … exactly what a heart attack is supposed to look like."

The family had requested the autopsy, perhaps because the death was so sudden, and somewhat unexpected. We knew his heart was weak; we knew he needed a stent. But no one thought he was going to suddenly die like that, certainly not me. *Don't you think you're getting better?!*

Now Mr. Lu's head was tipped back and his mouth hung slightly open; a trickle of clear-pink fluid ran from the corner of his mouth into his left ear. Beads of sweat sprinkled the side of his forehead and his left cheek in a strange distribution—not sweat, I realized after a moment, but condensation. A frozen body, thawing.

Tiny black nodules, like barnacles, ran in streaks over his skin in two places—one on his lower abdomen and one on his upper thigh. I wondered what they were. Sebhorreic keratosis, perhaps. I had never noticed them before, had never inspected his body closely enough to see them.

Over the center of his chest: faint pink and gray bruises, crevices and valleys where there should have been solid, flat bone underneath. An hour of vigorous chest compressions—while I was slicing my laps through the pool— had fractured his ribs. His sternum sank into his chest like a flattened football. Just to the left of the navel were a few spots of deep blue—bruises from his heparin shots. His penis lay brown and limp between pale thighs, under a shock of pubic hair, straight like grass. His toes were white.

Suddenly the pathologist had a knife in his hand and was slicing Mr. Lu's body open—not meticulously, layer by layer, like a surgeon, but aggressively, as though there was nothing to be heeded or protected. A deep V down the center of the chest, pointing at the belly button. He peeled back this triangular flap of skin, letting it rest on Mr. Lu's face. Then with a handheld electric saw, he buzzed through the ribs one at a time.

I reached out and patted Mr. Lu's forearm, as though to comfort him.

It's okay. I'm okay.

An hour later, the heart, large and floppy, lay on a plastic cutting board propped on Mr. Lu's knees. The pathologist took it in his gloved hands and slid his thumb under the pale pericardium, peeling it back to reveal smooth, glistening muscle underneath. Coronary vessels ran in shallow sulci, like rivers through valleys embedded in fatty foliage.

With a scalpel, he cut several crosswise slits down the length of the Left Anterior Descending artery. "Whoa, my god," he declared in mock dismay, as though receiving a bit of juicy gossip. "Look at that." He separated the slices with his fingertips to show me the vessel in cross-section. "Ninety-nine percent occlusion."

The walls of the artery were thick and white, like over-cooked macaroni. The central lumen was almost entirely blocked with white plaque: cholesterol.

"And what do you see there in the center?" he asked me, pointing. "That black pinpoint?"

"Clot?" I answered.

"Mm-hmm. Fresh blood clot. That is your cause of death right there. And let's see, the Left Main"—he sliced further up the heart. "Whoa! My god." Again he folded back the slices to show me. "See that? Total occlusion. You know what they call a total occlusion of the Left Main artery?"

I searched frantically for a diagnostic term from medical school, a pathologic word or phrase. "No, I ..."

"They call that 'The Widow-Maker.' "

We took a break. Dr. E removed his gloves and apron, stood there with his hands on his hips. Mr. Lu's organs were gathered in a red biohazard bag, which sat inside his hollow abdominal cavity. "We will just take a look at the brain," said Dr. E, "and then we're done. I'm going to get a soda. Nicky—you want anything? Diet Coke?"

"Yeah, sure, thanks."

He gestured to me. "You want anything?"

"No, I'm okay, thanks."

"You sure?"

While Dr. E went to the vending machine, Nicky cut an almond-shaped segment from the top of Mr. Lu's skull and began to pry at it with a metal spatula.

Dr. E returned and placed Nicky's Diet Coke on the counter. He stood sipping his Mountain Dew and pointed to Mr. Lu's brain, which was now exposed in his open skull. "See that? Some mild frontal lobe atrophy. Maybe he had a bit of dementia? Was he a bit slow?"

"Um, he was … no. Not slow," I said. "He … might have had some learning disabilities."

"Mmm. Maybe so. A little bit atrophied for his age. It's noticeable."

That night on the couch, Mo asked me, "How did it go?"

Images flashed through my head: pools of dark blood in an empty rib cage. Loops of bowel hanging from the pathologist's gloved hands, heavy and dripping like a brocaded skirt. Mr. Lu's face peeled down off of his skull, forehead to chin.

"It was … I mean it was awful to see him laid out on the table like that. But it was also good, in a way. It was good to see him again."

Suddenly my face was buried in his shoulder; his arms were around me. I clutched his shirt in my hands, pulling him into me. "I love you. Don't leave," I said, my tears warm and wet on his sleeve.

"I'm not leaving. I'm not going anywhere, ever."

In the middle of the night I lay next to Mo, trying to sleep. Our bodies were pressed together, his stomach on the small of my back, his legs tucked into the backs of my knees. Through the window, a cold breeze blew into the square, dark room. Suddenly I was confused. I smelled the morgue, hot metal and formaldehyde. His hand curled between my breasts, the hair poking from his T-shirt collar and his boxers, the soft lump of his penis, his warm breath. It was him. I scrambled away, kicking at the covers, finding the edge of the bed. Looking back, I saw Mo lift his face in the dark, questioning. Then he dropped his head to the pillow, saying nothing.

The truth is I don't really know her story.

Patients keep secrets without meaning to. They harbor them like sailboats on still water on a moonless night—unnoticed, unexpected. A fear of heights. A molesting uncle. A mother who committed suicide. Usually they don't tell me these things, because I don't ask. If I did, the answers could probably explain more than any CT scan or lumbar puncture ever could.

Only a few patients keep secrets deliberately, and those secrets are usually predictable, transparent. *How much alcohol do you drink? How many times have you been pregnant? Are you taking your blood pressure medicines?*

Ms. Kaur wasn't that type.

As with most of the patients I cared for during residency, what I knew of her story was only a collection of fragments, the bare minimum of medical details I gathered from her chart and my rushed history, plus a few additional pieces I picked up some mornings on my rounds. I didn't really know the sequence or the logic—if there was any—of how things unfolded before the day I met her. And now, of course, I'll never know.

The only person who could have put it all together for me was her sister, whom I will almost certainly never see again.

The difference between secrets and lies: that is one I have yet to pin down, in my medical practice or in life. Like most things, sometimes it's obvious. More often it's not.

Harpreet Kaur was a Punjabi Sikh. I don't know when she left India, but after many years in the U.S., she spoke only a few words of English. She lived with her sister Nuri, and Nuri's husband, in one of the small, mostly white working-class towns surrounding our hospital. Nuri was her primary caretaker, and as far as I know she always had been.

All the residents used to say Nuri was a saint, the way she cared so devotedly for her sister. She had a wise, soft face and calm, wide eyes. Her English was perfect, quiet; she was always ready, when asked, to provide her sister's up-to-date medication list from memory, a summary of her most recent and relevant health events, and any other information that could be of use to us. But she was never pushy with her information. She sat at her sister's bedside and waited, patiently, for the doctors to come with our questions.

Ms. Kaur had been blind since the age of eighteen. When I asked, Nuri explained that her sister had been blinded by a viral infection ("I think chicken pox?"). This was enough explanation for me. It also explained why, as a young woman from a small North Indian village, Ms. Kaur had never married.

At some point in her young life, Ms. Kaur must have contracted tuberculosis. A bronchoscopy report buried deep in her chart noted findings of severe restrictive lung disease "primarily due to post-tuberculosis fibrotic changes." In addition, she was found to have a moderate "obstructive component" to her airway disease, for which she had been prescribed a slew of daily inhalers and steroids. The cause of this chronic obstructive pulmonary disorder (COPD) was never really elucidated, as far as I could tell. In non-smoking women from the developing world, COPD is often chalked up to a lifetime of cooking over wood-burning stoves. But how could a blind woman have done any cooking over a wood-burning stove?

That was just Ms. Kaur's rotten luck: First the blindness. Then the TB. Then the severe post-TB restrictive lung disease, with a touch of COPD. Then, in her forties, Ms. Kaur was diagnosed with a diffuse large B cell lymphoma. That is when she really got sick. Her doctors tried chemotherapy, but she apparently "failed" after just one round, due to debilitating side effects.

The lymphoma was Stage IV—terminal—by the time I met Ms. Kaur during my intern year. The cancer was all over her body by then, but it was most obvious in her cervical lymph nodes: her neck and jaw were swollen with firm, golf-ball sized masses that made her look like a bird puffing up its throat in mating season. One night during my intern year, she came into the ER gasping for breath. She was intubated and sent to the ICU, where a senior resident cared for her. Eventually she was transferred to my service when she was almost well enough to go home.

It was one of many hospital admissions for Ms. Kaur that year. To her and Nuri, I was one of hundreds of doctors who cared for her. I doubt they would have remembered me if I hadn't spoken to her in my poor Hindi one morning, leaning close to her and holding her cool, ashen hand. "*Ji, kaise hain aj?*" ("How are you today?") For the first time, I saw her smile, a light turning on somewhere far behind her glazed, sunken eyes.

I suppose that for a brief moment, she thought one of her doctors might speak to her in her language. Which of course, I couldn't really do. She said something back to me in a flurry of enthusiastic words I didn't understand.

"How do you know Hindi?" Nuri asked me.

"My husband's family," I said proudly. "They are from India, too."

After that first overwhelming encounter as an intern, I met Ms. Kaur several times over the following three years. She was in and out of the hospital, always with difficulty breathing from a pneumonia or a flare of her COPD. When I saw her name on the admissions list in the ER, I always told the senior resident that they could send her to my service.

I liked Ms. Kaur, not just because she was a pleasant patient with few demands. I liked her smile, which I learned to coax out of her by pressing her hand or opening the curtains on a sunny day. I liked Nuri, too. Her calm, always slightly hoarse voice reminded me of Mo's grandmother. I recognized their intense familial devotion to one another; their trust in our medical expertise; the prayers they would mutter under their breath while waiting for the next doctor or nurse to approach the bedside.

One day as the senior resident on the critical care service, I was called to admit Ms. Kaur to the ICU in the middle of the night. She was in respiratory distress, wheezing and gasping for air. Nuri explained that her sister had just been discharged from a nearby hospital a few days before, after a three-week stay for a bad pneumonia. Now she seemed to have another pneumonia, and a COPD exacerbation, of course. She was worse than I'd ever seen her, sucking away on the BiPAP breathing mask in the ER, looking dangerously close to needing intubation. She was a sickly pale, her skin the color of powdered Ovaltine, dry and ashen. Her arms and legs were bone-thin, although her neck was thick and knobby as ever, a gnarled tree trunk stuck on the heaving scaffolding of her rib cage. As always her eyes were blank and her face was searching, her head craned slightly forward to catch the sounds and voices around her. But some of the urgency in her leaning body was gone. It was as though she had given up trying to understand, trying to see with her other senses. She was too tired.

We managed to avoid intubating her that night. Over the next several days she got a little better, then got a little worse again. Often at night she would become delirious. One night I sat with her for over an hour while she panted, her respiration rate in the forties. She was unresponsive to my voice; she just kept mumbling over and over, between frantic breaths, *"Waheguru. Waheguru. Waheguru"*—a mantra that invoked God. I rubbed her back, played some of Mo's grandmother's devotional *bhajans* on my phone for her, held her hand. Eventually I put the BiPAP mask back on her, despite her delirium. She gradually calmed and slept.

But she didn't get better. After several more days, the palliative care team was asked to step in. With their guidance, Ms. Kaur and Nuri agreed that the best thing was for her to go home with hospice. It was only a matter of time until her lungs gave out. She was, it turned out, loath to be intubated ever again. She would rather go home, she said, with morphine to ease her air hunger, than be placed on a ventilator while she waited for the cancer to take over her body from the inside out. At the age of fifty-five, Ms. Kaur was finally ready to die.

Arrangements were made for her to be discharged the following morning.

That night when I arrived, the daytime resident told me that Nuri had gone home for the evening. Her husband would be staying the night in the ICU with Ms. Kaur. I was glad Nuri was getting a chance to rest after all she'd been through that week. I figured Nuri's husband must know his sister-in-law well (she had lived in their home for years), and that he would be an adequate substitute to keep vigil for one night. As I walked by the room, I caught a glimpse of a tall, turbaned and bearded man standing beside Ms. Kaur's bed, watching her quietly.

About midnight, the nurse asked me to come to the room. Ms. Kaur was once more struggling to breathe. I examined her and decided to place her back on the BiPAP for the night, to keep her comfortable and let her sleep. After calling for the respiratory therapist, I introduced myself to Nuri's husband. "I'm the doctor taking care of her overnight," I explained. "And you must be her brother-in-law, right? Nuri's husband?"

He nodded. Something in his glance gave me pause. He opened his mouth as though he wanted to say something, but stopped. I proceeded to examine her while he looked on. I wasn't sure how involved he'd been, or how close he was to Ms. Kaur, but he seemed comfortable at her bedside. As I turned up the oxygen flowing through her mask and rubbed Ms. Kaur's back gently, I watched them interact for those few moments. He was kind, but direct: "Sit up now," he told her in English, then again in Punjabi. "Lean forward, you know that's how you breathe better." Similarly, she seemed vaguely irritated with him. Although I couldn't understand her response in her breathless Punjabi, I could tell exactly what she was saying from the way she clucked her tongue against the roof of her mouth and grimaced at him: *Oh stop telling me things I already know. Do you think I'm trying to make it more difficult?* This kind of casual irritation between two people, even under dire circumstances, bespoke an intimacy I hadn't expected between them.

After Ms. Kaur was comfortably on the BiPAP, her brother-in-law asked me to step out of the room with him for a moment.

"You know," he said, his voice hushed but calm, "this evening she told me she feels something is not right in her body. She says something has changed."

I nodded slowly, finding my footing in delicate territory. "Sometimes," I said, "people who are getting ready to die know before we do—before their doctors, before their families—when it's getting closer. To me, she looks about the same as she has the past couple of days. But to be on the safe side, perhaps I should call Nuri and ask her to come—"

He shook his head. "No, no. She doesn't need to come."

"Okay," I said. "But if you think she's changing overnight, or worsening, please don't hesitate to tell me. If Nuri wants to be here, I mean when—"

"No, she doesn't need to be here," he said, this time more emphatically. "I know what you are saying. But that's why I am here. I can take care of her. Anyway, she is okay right now. I just wanted to tell you that that's what she said."

"Okay," I said again. "Thanks for telling me."

I didn't know what to make of it.

Ms. Kaur made it through the night on the BiPAP. I hardly looked in on her. Her nurse, Monique, was vigilant and reliable. I knew I would hear from her if anything changed. When I did walk by the room, I always saw Nuri's husband sitting, calm but watchful, at the bedside.

Around 5 a.m., Monique appeared in the doctors' workroom. Her eyebrows were raised and the corners of her mouth tilted upward as though she were amused, or offended, or both. "Can I tell you something about Ms. Kaur?" she said.

Monique was a young African American traveler nurse from Georgia, with an accent thick and dripping like syrup, and a pretty, expressive face. She was easy to work with, not only because she had a good clinical sense of her patients, but because she was a good communicator. She hid nothing: her face and her tone of voice told you most everything you needed to know, even before she rattled off a set of vital signs or a lab result.

But that morning she seemed taken aback, almost mystified. I had no idea what she was going to tell me. "What is it?"

"You know the whole thing about Ms. Kaur bein' blind from chicken pox or whatever? Since she was eighteen?"

"Yeah?"

"Wait, so, can you even *get* blind from chicken pox really? 'Cause I never heard of that."

Honestly I had never heard of it either, but I bluffed. "Maybe from complications of chicken pox, or something."

"Oh, okay. Well anyway, so she been blind since she was eighteen and she never married. Or at least that's what I *thought,* that she was never married. Turns out she *was* married. To *that* guy in *there.*

"Wait, what? I thought that guy was—"

"You thought he was her sister's husband? I *know.* He *is.* I mean he's both. He and Ms. Kaur got married, and then they got divorced. Because she couldn't get pregnant. And *then* he *married* her *sister.*"

"You're kidding."

"That's what he told me."

"Jeeze. Just now he told you that?"

"Yeah, because I was going in to clean her, and I asked him if he wanted to, you know, step out the room or whatever. And he was like, 'No, it's alright, I'm her ex-husband, it's fine.' And I was like, 'You're her *what?!*

I thought you was her brother-in-law,' and he was like, 'I'm both.'"

"He *said* that?!"

"Yeah, and then he explained it all to me."

"Jeeze."

"I know, right?"

"That's so weird. And isn't it also still kind of weird that he stayed in the room while you cleaned her and stuff? I mean it's not like they're *still* married."

"I *know!*"

For a moment I caught myself. We were gossiping like teenagers. But I'd been up all night with no one to talk to, just my computer and a bunch of sedated patients, their ventilators beeping and sighing. I went on. "I mean, you'd think maybe she would want some kind of *privacy*."

"That's exactly what I was thinking!" Monique's eyebrows shot up. "But I was actually thinking that before, just in the way he was talking to her. Like, he was kinda tellin' her what to do and stuff?"

"Really? Huh. I noticed that too, but I guess I thought he seemed ... caring."

"Oh yeah he *cares* about her, you can tell that. I just mean—I don't know. I don't want to be judging

any kind of culture or any kind of man. I don't even
know what kind of culture they are, but—"

"They're Punjabi Indians," I said. "Sikhs."

"Oh. How'd you know that?"

I paused. "They're from the same part of India as
my husband's family," I said.

"Oh." She glanced at me then, and I thought I
could see her thinking, *God. Well what does SHE put up
with from HER husband?*

There was a silence between us for a moment, just
the hum and the beeps of the ICU behind us. I thought
about Ms. Kaur. I saw her life with a new and profound
sense of unfairness: the burden of one disease and one
impairment after another, the way she depended on her
sister to take care of her in a foreign country, in a dark,
hostile world. And all along, she'd been living in her
sister's home while her sister was married to her ex-
husband. I thought of Nuri and her selfless devotion to
her sick, blind sister. ("She's a saint," we all said.) Maybe
the secret didn't matter. I didn't doubt Nuri's motives,
and I felt sure Ms. Kaur didn't, either. But I felt I was
seeing something I should have seen before, something
I should have known, from my own experience and
my own marriage: that love, particularly the love of
families, is never simple. It is always complex, entangled.
Everything touches everything. The love of our families

is touching us every second if we let ourselves notice it. And as beautiful and necessary as love is, there is nothing about it, not a single centimeter of it, that isn't raw and painful.

And now, this morning, Harpreet Kaur was going home to her family, to die.

"Poor Ms. Kaur," I whispered.

"Mm-hmm." Monique took in a deep breath and let it out. "You know, I don't care what anyone says. I don't care who you are or what country you come from. I think all women feel the same things."

I looked up at her.

"You know?" she said.

"Yeah," I said. "Yeah, I think so, too."

TWENTY-FOUR WEEKS

MOST LEARNING IN MEDICINE is improvisational. Doctors often talk about it as though it is a game: "Fake it till you make it." Pretend you know what you're doing, until one day you do. They don't say this under their breath. Various attending physicians at all stages of my training gave me the "Fake it till you make it" line as though it were the best advice they had to offer, and probably it was.

My co-residents seemed comfortable with this approach, rising to the occasion, doing the best they could until they gradually got better and better. But I writhed under this mantra like a spider in a draining tub. I am too much of a perfectionist, too sensitive. Not to say that my colleagues were sloppy or obtuse. But they didn't seem to need or want the kind of guidance

I craved: step-by-step, intentional instruction. Watching Denise Winters thrash against piles of blankets on a hospital bed. Hearing the roaring silence on the other side of the stethoscope. Clenching my jaw as Dr. K pointed to that floating embryo, his ultrasound probe still stuffed between the patient's legs. These were the moments when I wanted someone to act as a buffer against my inexperience, a cushion to keep the patients safe from my mistakes. I suppose what I really wanted was to be protected from my own mistakes.

Twenty-four weeks is a critical point in obstetrics. Known as the point of viability, it is the gestational age at which the fetus is capable, at least theoretically, of surviving outside the womb. "Survival," however, doesn't necessarily mean "meaningful life," life without the support of technology, or even a life of more than a few days. Still, this threshold has become paramount in medical ethics and law. A fetus that leaves the uterus before viability is called a miscarriage or a stillbirth. Even if there is a heartbeat, there is no effort at medical resuscitation, because these efforts would be futile and cause unnecessary suffering. (This reasoning represents one of the most—if not the most—profoundly unsettled and unsettling areas of medical ethics.) After the point of viability, around twenty-four weeks, what emerges from the womb is called a baby. Hospitals and parents, if they so choose, can spend huge amounts of effort and money to keep these babies alive.

By this same reasoning, twenty-four weeks (or, in legal terms, the "point of viability" as determined by a physician) is the legal limit of elective abortion in California and many other states. Because this point is the medical threshold for administering neonatal life support, many experts feel it is a reasonable cutoff for electively terminating a pregnancy.

In truth, viability is more complicated than this. The nuances can be hard to appreciate unless you've seen a baby born at twenty-four weeks: weighing less than a pound, its skin still translucent, lungs sticky and wet and unable to expand, eyeballs starved for oxygen (or sometimes poisoned by too much oxygen). Unable to breathe, eat, or cry, and likely to be permanently blind, writhing on the warmer under bright lights and wires and heating coils, it is more like a primitive nervous system than a human being.

I am exactly twenty-four weeks pregnant today.

If I were comforted by the idea of "viability," I would breathe a sigh of relief right about now. I would feel that I'd made it past some turning point into a zone of safety and certainty. But I am not comforted at all.

At our appointment last week, the obstetrician asked, "Are you feeling the baby moving?"

"Yes," I said. "I feel it every day now."

"But I still can't feel it," Mo said, surprising us both.

The doctor smiled. "No, of course not. First, she feels the baby inside of her. Then later, you feel it too. You can only feel it on the outside, through her."

It seems like an obvious thing, but it was nice to hear it said aloud.

It is early fall. The mornings have turned cold again, even though the days are still bright, hot, and dry. I am waking up earlier and earlier—six o'clock, five o'clock—writing once again by the warmth of the space heater and the glow of the lamp, while Mo sleeps inside and the garden rests in its dark shadows. Most mornings now I sit in my armchair instead of at my desk, raising my feet to ease the ache at the small of my back. Curled up here, I can feel an occasional kicking and rolling inside of me, something comfortable and at the same time restless, like a kitten in my lap. Sometimes the real cat, seeing the light on, meows at the door, asking to join me. She has to drape herself across my knees—she's run out of room at the tops of my thighs.

This morning, instead of remembering the babies I've seen born at twenty-four weeks (perhaps because it's too painful and terrifying to think of them), I am remembering a twenty-four-week abortion, the only one I have ever seen.

In my final year of medical school, I was given a coveted medical student spot working in our university's hospital-based abortion clinic. As the one medical student, I was surrounded by and integral to the workings of the clinic: I did most of the pre-operative ultrasounds, dating the pregnancies to determine whether and when the woman could have her procedure. I watched the counselors speak with the patients, prepared their consent forms, performed physical exams, and learned to insert osmotic dilators. During that month, I performed very few abortions myself—maybe half a dozen early, simple procedures, always closely watched by a family planning fellow or attending physician. Nevertheless, it was the beginning of my training as an abortion provider.

One afternoon a sixteen-year-old girl appeared at the door with her mother. They had driven from Nevada, arriving at five o'clock on a Friday, just as the clinic was closing. She was pretty in the way of a healthy teenage girl: plump and athletic, she was a volleyball player from a working-class family. Her straw-blond hair was thick and straight, falling over her shoulders, and her eyes flashed with a certain kind of excitement; I imagined it had to do with her being a child in what she knew was a very adult situation.

I brought her into a dark room. On the table, she lifted her shirt to reveal her bulging abdomen, her navel surrounded by a ring of fine golden hairs, which flattened and glistened under the slick coat of ultrasound gel. She told me she and her boyfriend had had sex only a few times. Sometime last summer, her period had stopped. Now it was January. On the black and white screen that was a window into her uterus, I immediately saw that the heart was bigger than a flicker; it was a distinct organ of four chambers, beating its rhythm beneath a white-picket ribcage. I measured the diameter of the fetal skull and the length of a single femur, smaller than a toothpick, but still larger than any I'd measured before.

I called the doctor into the room. She agreed with the measurements: twenty-four weeks exactly.

Unfortunately the abortion could not happen today, the doctor explained to the girl and her mother. Her cervix would have to be opened first with osmotic dilators; this would take at least twenty-four hours. If she wanted to proceed, the only option was to inject a medication directly through her abdominal wall into the fetus's beating heart. The medicine would be effective immediately. "The fetus will stop growing," the doctor explained. In the meantime, we would place dilators to stretch her cervix over two nights. When she returned to the clinic, a repeat ultrasound would still show a twenty-four-week size fetus (instead of twenty-four weeks and two days), allowing for a legal abortion.

"Do you understand?"

The girl nodded. I watched her climb onto the exam table as I held the ultrasound probe and the doctor drew up the syringe. Her face was calm and closed, and I thought I had never seen such a brave person in my life.

I had always liked the idea of "family planning" as a medical specialty. That was why I had applied for a one-month rotation in the abortion clinic in the first place. But it was just an idea: a vague belief in "a woman's right to choose" and a general clinical interest in women's reproductive health.

After that day, that girl, and that particular confluence of circumstances—her arrival at the eleventh hour, in the twenty-fourth week, her bravery and resolve, and the opportunities and choices reopened to her by that one choice we allowed her to make—the work of family planning became something more tangible and urgent to me. It was the work of unraveling a complex knot of circumstance to reveal a beginning and an ending, a continuous thread of meaning, an arc. It was the work of storytelling, but not merely as a writer. As a family planning doctor, I could help a woman write her own story.

Now, instead of thinking of that moment in terms of the "viability" of a fetus, I find myself thinking about the point of viability in the life of a woman, and of a young doctor. That procedure, even though I only watched it, represented a threshold in that girl's life, and also in my training—a critical juncture. Up until then, I'd had plenty of doubts about my own survival. But that evening in the abortion clinic, after everyone else had gone home and it was just me, the doctor, the girl, and her mother, I found a clearer vision for my future, and a resolution to finish what I'd started.

But as with those tiny twenty-four-week babies strapped to their machines and monitors, blind and struggling, resolution and hope were not enough to get me through. I think of that first year of residency, those impossibly long days and nights at the hospital, the bitter fights with Mo and the alienation from my better self, and I wonder how I survived to the next turning point, when, in my second year of residency, shortly after that talk with Dr. Brennan, I began performing abortions again.

The bulk of my abortion training took place outside the walls of our residency hospital and clinic, where relatively few abortions were performed on any given day. Instead I was trained in Planned Parenthood clinics as part of the TEACH partnership, a program whose goal is to help primary care doctors integrate abortion care into their practice.

TEACH trainers are family physicians who believe in increasing access to abortion for all women by teaching other family doctors to perform the procedure. They have been trained in a holistic model of practice and teaching, which is not just about performing a safe abortion, but about understanding the context and controversy around abortion care in the U.S., addressing structural barriers that prevent women from accessing abortion, and helping primary care doctors become leaders in reproductive health.

The program's approach to procedural training is methodical and thorough. I had performed hundreds of gynecologic procedures and delivered nearly a hundred babies by that point in my residency. I had even performed those few abortions as a medical student. But on my very first TEACH training day, in my second year of residency, my only responsibility was to watch and learn.

I was told to arrive an hour before the clinic began. My trainer that day, Sarah McNeil, was the medical director of the TEACH program. She sat with me in an office and talked me through the first few chapters of the TEACH workbook, which I had been asked to read in advance. We reviewed equipment, techniques, and clinical scenarios. She asked me questions to test my knowledge, and she answered my questions on points I didn't understand. I wasn't thrown in and told to "get my hands in there" and "learn by doing," as we were in the hospital. Instead, when the first patient was ready, I followed Dr. McNeil into the room.

It was more or less what I expected: a clean, bare space; a green vinyl procedure table with two metal footrests; a stool for the doctor. A counter stocked with supplies and small suction devices (called MVA or manual vacuum aspirators). An electric vacuum aspirator (EVA), with its clear plastic tubing and glass jars, in the corner. Boxes of plastic gloves, a red sharps container bolted to the wall, an ultrasound machine on wheels.

On the table sat a young woman in her early thirties, with pale skin and dark brown hair pulled into a ponytail. She hugged her knees under the paper drape, her face open and calm. She looked prepared, or maybe resigned. I knew from the chart that she was carrying a pregnancy of about seven weeks. She had two children at home, she told us, one less than a year old. She had never resumed her birth control after having her second child, thinking she would be protected from pregnancy while she was breastfeeding. It was a story I would come to know well. She was, in many ways, a typical abortion patient.

Dr. McNeil introduced herself, then motioned toward me. "This is Dr. Henneberg," she said. "We'll be working together today." She sat down and began talking to the patient. I stood at her side, listening, never saying a word. Then I watched as she completed the entire procedure. I never once touched this young woman with my gloved hands.

Over time, Dr. McNeil and a team of about six other TEACH doctors taught me, step by step, how to perform a first-trimester abortion. Gradually I eased into the doctor's stool, placing the speculum, injecting lidocaine, dilating the cervix. With time and repetition—I did about two hundred abortions in the TEACH program—the procedure began to embed itself into my muscle memory, my hands undertaking the movements without conscious thought. When I slow down and think through the steps now, I can still hear the voices of my teachers ringing in my ears, and I can almost feel the corresponding areas of my brain light up as on a functional MRI: the palms of my hands tingle at the thought of those movements I know so well, the pull of my wrist, the pressure under my knuckles. Over the past five years those movements have become as familiar as a pen in my hand moving across the page, as the click of these keystrokes under my fingertips.

It begins and ends in the space between your hands.

With one hand, you reach inside to find the cervix. The vagina—contrary to the posters on the walls of doctors' offices, but true to any woman's experience of sexual intercourse—is not a hollow tunnel, but a closed space that must be pried open. In medicine the term is a "potential space." A penis, a finger, a speculum, a drop of blood, a baby's head—any of these things must push their way through the vagina, creating a passage in or out. In this case, it is your right hand—two gloved fingers smeared with gel—that finds its way gently back to the cervix, the door to the uterus.

With the left hand pressing on the lower abdomen, you find the firm bulge at the top of the uterus, called the fundus. With some pressure, you can cradle the uterus between your hands to get a sense of its size and shape and subtle tilt within the body. It can be the size of a lemon (not pregnant, or barely pregnant) to the size of a cantaloupe (twenty-four weeks), bulging just above the navel. It can tilt upward toward the ceiling or back toward the table. It is a secret organ, but not a fickle one. Built of thick muscle and pulsing with a network of blood vessels (ultimately using about one third of the blood in the woman's body at any given moment in the third trimester), the uterus is built to be strong and resilient.

Looking inside the vagina, again prying open that potential space with the speculum, you look down the tunnel you've created to see the cervix, a pink doughnut with a snug opening at its center. The cervical canal is another potential space, but this one cannot be nudged open with just a finger. It must be stretched, either overnight with expanding dilators, or in the moment, using a series of metal rods. This is one of the trickiest parts of an otherwise straightforward procedure: to learn how much pressure—sometimes an enormous amount of pressure—you must apply against the cervix with each progressively larger dilator. It is an act of force executed with the touch of utmost control. It can take all the strength in your shoulder and wrist, but you must be as gentle as though you were painting a hollowed Easter egg. One by one, the dilators push through. The cervix does—and will, eventually—open like a door. But if your dilator slips through the cervix too quickly, or at a slightly wrong angle, you will perforate, poking a hole through that muscular uterine wall, opening a passageway between uterus and abdominal cavity and potentially causing severe bleeding and infection. So you must be patient with the cervix. You must let it open on its own terms.

When you have passed the last dilator, the next step is the suction, the removal of the embryo or fetus through a thin plastic tube, the cannula. The size of the pregnancy determines how wide you must open the cervix to make room for the appropriate size cannula. A 6-flex cannula (a thin, flexible rubber tube) is just large enough to remove a six-week pregnancy. A "12-rigid" or "12-flex" can remove a twelve-week pregnancy. And so forth until about sixteen weeks, after which the pregnancy is too large to remove through a tube, and must be removed in pieces, with forceps—a technically much more difficult procedure called a D&E.

You can aspirate by feel, or you can use the ultrasound to guide your movements: if her anatomy is unusual, if you're unsure of what you sense with your hands, or if it is a later pregnancy where the risk of leaving something behind (or perforating the uterus with your instruments) is greater. Over time, you will become more comfortable with the sensations, and your hands will become your eyes. You learn to feel the pregnancy against the smooth wall of the uterus, with the tip of the cannula working for you like an extension of your body, one long finger. You will even feel as the pregnancy tissue whips through the cannula and down into the suction chamber, and the immediate response of the uterus afterward—remember, it is pure muscle—to clamp down and expel whatever blood and endometrium is left behind. After removing the cannula, you should reach inside with a clean glove, find the cervix, repeat the bimanual exam. You will feel that the uterus has contracted; it is a tight, tiny rock between your hands.

Now it is time to leave the room, just for a few minutes. The patient will stay on the table, so you switch off the procedure lamp and tug the paper drape down between her thighs. Maybe lay a hand on her knee for a moment; often she is trembling from the weight of her legs and her emotions. "I'll be right back. I'm going to make sure it's finished." Take your little metal dish or glass bottle to the lab, run it under cold water through a fine strainer, and watch as the bright red blood and dark clots wash away. What's left behind is a handful of clumpy tissue, mostly lining from the wall of the uterus.

Sift through these clumps in a Plexiglas dish, held over a light, and you will find the pregnancy. At ten to twelve weeks, it's obvious what you're looking for: tiny hands and legs, a string of vertebrae, the translucent eggshell of the fetal skull called the calvarium. But most abortions occur before a fetal body has formed. At five to eight weeks, all you will see is the gestational sac, a membrane so delicate and transparent it looks like a wisp of cloud in the sky. But press this little membrane under your gloved fingertip, and you will feel something stronger than you could ever have imagined. No matter how hard you pull and press on it, it will not tear. It is enough to make you wary of what you have just done—something unnatural, yes, and nature has put up tremendous barriers to resist it. But nature is not always a friend of man or woman, and now you, with your little plastic tube and hand-held suction device, have overcome it.

When you return to the room, you will tell the woman, "The abortion is over. You're no longer pregnant. Nothing about the procedure will affect your ability to get pregnant in the future."

And most of the time she will look up at you, with or without tears in her eyes, and say, "Thank you."

And you should tell her, "You're welcome."

The difference between my abortion training and the rest of my medical training was that in the abortion clinic, I felt safe. It wasn't just the methodical, highly supervised learning model of the TEACH program that gave me that sense of safety. It had to do with the work itself, the patients, and what they needed from me as their doctor.

For the most part, by the time a woman lies down on the table, naked below the waist, covered in a paper drape, she has made a decision. From that point on, the interaction between doctor and patient tends to fit into a familiar template: There she is on the table, with all the difficulty of her decision (or liberation, or relief, or all of those things) bundled tightly inside of her. She has been given plenty of time with the clinic counselors to ask questions, to sort through any shame, sadness, or ambivalence. The message is not said but implied: Figure it out now, before you get to the procedure room, because the doctor's time is valuable. She has been counseled about pain and anxiety, given relaxation techniques (wiggle your toes, breathe in deeply through your nose and out through your mouth), and given a dose of I.V. sedative and narcotic. She has been told that it is okay to cry, but not to scream; she is reminded that there are women waiting their turn on the other side of the wall.

My job in that room is to treat her with respect and dignity, to confirm that she is sure of her decision, and then to perform a procedure that is as safe, short, and painless as possible. It is not exactly an easy job, but it is a clear one.

In the beginning it was the clarity of the job—and the clarity of its boundaries—that made me feel safe. Although I told myself I could identify with the woman on the table, that I could just as easily be in her shoes, I didn't really believe that. I believed I was safe in my world of black-and-white, a world of smart choices, choices that kept me from ever having to be the one with my feet in the stirrups. The gray area was where my patients were. The pregnant women. The mothers.

These were the women—like the sixteen-year-old girl from Nevada—to whom I had been drawn from the beginning, the women who had the most reason to feel vulnerable and afraid. I wanted to offer them safety and agency in their lives, to help them rewrite the story.

But whose story was I writing? Who was I really protecting?

Going through my papers recently, I came across a short essay, "What I Like About Being an Abortion Provider." From the date, I can tell I wrote it just a few months into my second year of residency, when I had just begun my abortion training with TEACH.

"What I like about being an abortion provider"

As I get closer to my final year of residency, people have started asking me what I want to do after I graduate. I pause and consider whether to give an honest answer. "Well," I say, "I really like doing abortions."

This answer can be a conversation stopper.

"What do you like about doing abortions?" my friend Angie said, and I knew I'd offended her. Angie isn't the only one of my friends who's had an abortion. They all know that abortions are a part of my training. But I realized too late that to say that I "like" this work may sound cruel, even sadistic to her. She remembers her own abortion as something emotionally and physically traumatic.

It must make it even more painful to think of an abortion doctor—her own friend—enjoying the procedure.

What is there to like about performing abortions?

Technically, it's a simple procedure. I happen to think there is nuance and beauty in exploring the uterus, a three-dimensional space that one cannot see with one's own eyes. (Some nights after a day of abortion training, I've had dreams of cave-diving in the dark, using my hands to navigate vast chambers and hidden passageways.) But of course this uterine-exploring experience is part of many obstetrical and gynecologic procedures. Plenty of gynecologists will declare that a manual aspiration is nothing more than a glorified endometrial biopsy— and mechanically speaking, this is true.

The joy and the challenge of the work, for me, begins the moment I walk into the room, meet the patient's eyes, and call her by her name. Every move I make from that moment on—every word, every gesture—is intentional. I am, almost invariably, meeting a human being in her deepest moment of shame, fear, and often sadness. My job is not just to end her pregnancy safely; it is to ease her suffering, so that she leaves the room thinking, at the very least, that it wasn't as bad as she'd feared.

Every doctor knows that to ease suffering is not the same as relieving pain. It is not something we accomplish by applying lidocaine to the cervix, or by using warm gel on the speculum, or even playing soothing music in the background. More than anything, we ease suffering with our words and our touch.

The more abortions I perform and the more comfortable I become with the procedure itself, the more I realize that this is the real challenge: to ease suffering with my words and my touch. While my usual comforting phrases feel right with ninety-nine percent of women, occasionally they sound hollow to my ears, or the woman is confused by my instructions, or my gentle touch startles and unnerves her. So I observe each woman carefully in the brief time I have in the room with her, watching for clues in her face and body, experimenting and tailoring my words and my touch to meet her where she is in that moment. I do this with the same level of attention that I give to the bimanual exam, when I use the information I gather with my fingertips to subtly adjust the tilt of the speculum or the angle of a dilator, fitting the curves of her body, that invisible space of her uterine cavity.

As I learn to become a better abortion doctor, I must also learn how to talk about the work I'm doing—whether I aim to hide it, defend it, or explain it. One thing is certain: I can't walk around telling everyone who asks that I like (I would even say love) providing abortions. But to my friends who ask, and to other friends and colleagues I trust, this is what I can say: When I perform one abortion, I provide a service for a woman that will change the story of her life. And with my own words and touch—my ability to comfort and reassure her, to ease her suffering—I can actually write the first page of that story with her.

Reading it now makes me cringe. The stuff about the poor "suffering woman," and me, the heroic doctor, there to save her and ease her suffering. It's all there, that sense of clarity and safety that I clung to so desperately, as black and white as the ink on the page.

After I wrote it, I sent the essay to Sarah McNeil, the TEACH director, asking her if she had any suggestions for where I might publish it.

"It's nice," she said. "But I'm not sure if it's publishable. We all already know this stuff, you know? It's all been said before, many times."

Probably she was right. But I seethed with bitterness at her response, her misunderstanding of my intentions. Who did she mean by "we"? The abortion community? The Society for Family Planning? This wasn't the audience I was writing for. I didn't want to be one of those doctors who occasionally published a piece on the *New England Journal* "Perspectives" page and called herself a writer. I wanted to be a real writer, to write for other people, people who read books, not medical journals. People like Angie, who had had abortions, and people who hadn't. People who didn't realize that an abortion could be anything other than a grisly, shameful, tragic thing.

Anyway, even if, as Dr. McNeil said, the point of the essay was nothing special, I thought my ability to put it into words was. I had hoped my writing would help me stand out to my abortion trainers at TEACH, so they would take an interest in me and perhaps help me find more training opportunities, or even a job after I graduated.

But apparently my compassion and my writing were not going to be enough. I began to understand that what was going to matter most were my training and skills. Like any area of medicine, abortion care must be safe, efficient, and solvent. The doctor must be there not only to make the patients feel cared for, but to complete procedures quickly and skillfully. It wasn't enough to be passionate and articulate about the work. I needed to do procedures. Lots of them.

THIRTY WEEKS

I KEEP ALL THE baby things stacked in a corner of the garage: high chair, car seat, bassinet, stroller. Hidden under a white sheet, they make a strange, mountainous form next to our bikes and Costco packs of toilet paper.

Mo went in there the other day to get a light bulb. "Isn't that a bit much?" he said.

"What?" I said, looking up. I was reading on the couch, my feet stretched out in front of me and propped on two pillows, my book resting on my belly.

I could see him choosing his words. "I know you don't want all the baby stuff all over the house. But ... ah ... the sheet. It's kind of morbid. It kind of looks like, you know, like somebody died."

I shrugged, turning back to my book. "It'll just have to look that way for now."

Later that same day, my friend Toby called me. She and her wife, Kersh, have been trying to conceive for four years with donor sperm. During that time, she's watched a dozen of her friends get pregnant and give birth.

She was breathless on the phone. "Chrissy," she said. "I have news."

Toby is a violinist, opera singer, and private music teacher in San Francisco. I've seen her teach. She is animated and encouraging, the kind of music teacher who throws open the door and welcomes each student as though they're her favorite, squeezing their little shoulders in a hug. At the end of the lesson, she sends them out with a triumphant pat on the back and a plea to get in their thirty minutes of daily practice. Each one of those kids probably believes they could perform at the Met if they wanted to.

"I'm pregnant," she said.

For half an hour, I did nothing but congratulate Toby and listen as she recounted the details. She'd just gotten the result of her second blood draw, which showed a rising beta-HCG level—the pregnancy hormone. She is barely in her fifth week, too early even for an ultrasound. "We're naming her Juniper!" she announced.

While we talked, I paced the backyard, feeling the now-familiar movements under my ribcage, looking down at my feet in the grass, barely visible beyond my bulging abdomen.

Toby and I haven't talked much the past six months. I haven't told her I'm pregnant. I didn't tell her on the phone that afternoon, either. Toby is a soprano; she likes to be the center of attention. I didn't want to take away from her triumphant moment.

Actually, I've hardly told anyone. Our parents and sisters, of course, some close friends, and some acquaintances I've made swimming laps at the pool (impossible to hide it there). More people are starting to notice, though. Over the past few weeks, my colleagues at work have started asking me. Even my loose scrub tops now make a conspicuous tent over my belly.

At first I was nervous about what my abortion patients would say when I started showing. But they always expressed genuine happiness for me, even in the midst of their own difficult decisions. "Girl, you are going to *love* that baby," one mother of three said to me before her procedure. Another woman, nineteen years old and ending her first pregnancy, smiled at me through her tears. "It's your time," she said.

Since sharing her news, Toby has been calling me almost every day. She had a third blood draw, then an ultrasound, which showed a yolk sac and an early fetal pole. She has questions for me about these images and the life growing inside her. "We saw her doing little trampoline jumps in there already! She's so active! I know they say you can't feel kicks until twenty weeks, but I swear I can feel something. Don't you think that's possible? That I can feel her?"

I finally told her my own news, hoping she wouldn't be annoyed at me for holding out on her. But she was ecstatic.

"Oh! Chrissy! Pregnant together! We're pregnant together! Oh, this is the best. The best! They'll be like sisters, only six months apart, right? Oh, Chrissy I can't wait. I can't wait, I can't wait!"

I have to say, her enthusiasm is sort of infectious. I can imagine Toby with her students, praising them as they saw away on their little violins. It's made me resolve to be more enthusiastic with my prenatal patients when they ask me, *Do you think everything will be okay?* I always hedge on questions like that, reluctant to make any promises. I see a pregnant woman and, in my mind, I don't see a baby. I see Kaitlyn.

But maybe what a woman needs—or most women, anyway—is to be told that everything is going to be okay. Even if, every once in a while, that turns out not to be true. It has certainly helped me, hearing Toby talk about it like that: a sure thing, a certainty. Juniper.

I have started sleeping on my side with a pillow between my legs, my hips stacked one on top of the other. When Mo crawls into bed next to me, he wraps one arm across my chest, his hand resting between my breasts and the bulge of my belly. His other hand touches my top hip. My back curves into him. Already I can feel the shape of our family forming.

Even now, I find myself sitting here in my pink armchair, imaging it—a little person I'll hold in my arms in just a few weeks, the weight of it off my pelvic bones and into my arms, a living, beautiful thing.

"Do you think," Toby said later, "that your little baby sort of helped usher little Juniper into being? You know, I've had so many pregnant friends over the past four years, but I've never had this feeling before. Maybe because you're one of my very closest friends, somehow I just feel like, I don't know, like the universe created our little babies to come into the world together."

In order to perform a second-trimester abortion—
called a D&E or "dilation and evacuation"—I need
the cervix to open considerably wider than in first-
trimester procedures. Because the fetal parts are larger
and more rigid, they cannot fit through a small plastic
cannula. Instead I use forceps, which look like slender
salad tongs, to remove the fetus. I must have enough
room to maneuver the handles, opening and closing
them to grasp the fetal parts and pull them from the
uterus. In order to dilate the cervix enough, the patient
must come to the clinic twice: once to have osmotic
dilators placed in her cervix, and again twenty-four
to forty-eight hours later for her abortion procedure.
The osmotic dilators look like tiny tampons and act
like sponges, relying on the biologic principle of
osmosis. Stuffed inside the tight cervical canal and left
there overnight, they absorb fluid from the cervix and
vagina, expanding and stretching the cervical canal in
the process.

In medical school, an excellent nurse practitioner
taught me how to insert osmotic dilators. Her name

was Mindy. I remember her as middle-aged, tall and slim with gray hair and light blue eyes. She explained her approach: "The first thing she needs to do is to open her legs so I can get to her vagina and her cervix. This is incredibly difficult for some women. I never use the words 'spread your knees' or 'spread your legs,' even though that's exactly what I need her to do. Too many women have heard those words in a situation of violence or threat. And no matter how long it takes, I never apply even the tiniest bit of pressure to the insides of her thighs. I will lose her trust before I've even started."

The placement of osmotic dilators can be very painful. The cervix is a snug space, a potential space, and when anything squeezes through it, in or out, the uterus cramps in response, causing spasms like a charley horse deep in the groin. When I was learning the procedure, many of the women cried out in pain—especially those who had never given birth, whose cervix had never yielded to any force. At first, I couldn't stand it. I felt I was torturing them, that I must be doing something wrong, and I would call for Mindy to take over. Despite her gentle demeanor and soft, high voice, she was resolute in the most difficult procedures. She knew how to talk to patients and transfer some of her confidence to them. "You can do this. You've started now. You can tell me to stop anytime, and I will. But I believe you can do this. There's nothing to be afraid of." After a while, I learned to talk to them the same way—firm but kind, unwavering in my belief in their strength. I knew it was good training if I ever wanted to be an abortion doctor myself.

A few months before finishing my residency, I drove to Los Angeles to see about a possible job. I was to spend three days working with Rebecca Sanders, the medical director of a group of high-volume family planning clinics based in Southern California. She wanted to observe my procedural skills and potentially get me "trained up" to work for her after graduation. There was an opening for an abortion doctor to work one day a week in a clinic in Modesto, in California's Central Valley.

Residency graduation was a few months away. Finally on the brink of finishing my training, I was feeling desperate for some kind of affirmation, someone to tell me I was good at something, that they would invest in me. More than anything, I wanted to find work as an abortion provider.

It was early March. I left in the morning, driving down Interstate 5, the same route Mo and I used to take driving to college. It had rained that weekend. The fields and surrounding hills were brilliant green. The fruit orchards were erupting in blossoms, a halo of pink petals surrounding each tree.

I arrived after dark and stayed with friends that night. In the morning I met Dr. Sanders at her clinic in Long Beach. "Call me Rebecca," she said, gripping my hand. She was beautiful. She wore a pair of gray scrubs and no makeup, her dark, curly hair pulled back in a low ponytail. Her skin was olive-colored and clear, and although she had the common look of chronic exhaustion that I knew so well among my colleagues—bags under her eyes, a slight hunch to her neck and shoulders—there was a bounce in her step as she led me to the morning huddle before the day's first procedure. As she began talking to the team gathered around her—medical assistants, a recovery nurse, a nurse anesthetist, and several counselors—I could see she was energized by this moment, and by the day ahead. Sixty abortions were on the schedule. More than thirty would be second-trimester procedures (D&Es) on women who were already lined up in the waiting room with osmotic dilators inside of them.

Rebecca briefed the staff on the day's schedule, introduced me and some other staff in training, and gave a few concise clinical updates, including a mention of Zika virus and the importance of screening pregnant women for recent travel to Latin America. ("Only women who are continuing their pregnancies, of course.") Her staff listened, quiet and attentive. The whole thing took less than five minutes.

"Alright—break!" The day began.

Rebecca pulled me into her office. "Chris, before we get going: we have a lot of procedures to get through. It's an average volume for me, but average days are busy here. I recognize that after doing thousands and thousands of abortions, I can seem sort of … desensitized. It's not that I don't recognize what a significant moment this is for most of these women. I do. But I'm here to help them. I have to move fast. You'll see. If at any time you need to step out, or sit down, or whatever—just do it. Okay?"

"Got it," I said.

We entered the first operating room.

The patient was on the table in a gown, the medical assistant standing at her side. Rebecca placed an IV in her arm while she gave the patient a little pep talk—a routine I would hear more than a hundred times over the next three days. "This is a very short, very safe procedure," she told her. "Do you have any questions for me before we get started?" Usually there were none.

"Okay my dear, now we're going to get your legs up and over the bars and put your feet in the footrests. It's a big uncomfortable stretch, but then we're going to put you to sleep, and you won't be in this position when you wake up. This is your nurse anesthetist, she's going to put you to sleep. We'll see you in about ten minutes, okay?"

As the milky white Propofol rushed into the woman's arm, Rebecca was already at the foot of the table, placing a tray and a big metal bowl between the patient's legs, pulling on a pair of surgical gloves. She watched for the sign that the patient was out: her leg muscles suddenly slackening and her bottom sinking into the table. At that moment, she pushed the paper drape from between the woman's legs and plunged her fingers inside the vagina. She pulled out a soggy piece of gauze, then five swollen osmotic dilators that she plopped onto the tray next to her. Then her hand went back into the vagina, while her other hand pressed down on her abdomen so she could feel the shape and size of the uterus between her hands. She pulled her hand out, placed a weighted speculum in the vagina, hooked the anterior lip of the cervix with a tenaculum. All this took a matter of seconds. Then she placed a large cannula through the cervix, passing through the internal os (the inner opening of the cervix into the uterus), and asked the assistant to turn on the suction. Clear yellow fluid rushed through the cannula into the vacuum tube—she had broken the amniotic sac. Suction off. Cannula out. Forceps. Watching alternately the cervix and the ultrasound screen, she began pulling fetal parts out: calvarium, arms, spine and thorax, one leg, then another, then the pillowy placenta. Another spin with the cannula to remove any remaining uterine lining. Tenaculum off, another bimanual exam, speculum out. Bloody gloves stripped off and thrown onto the table, and she walked out of the room.

After a second, her head peered around the edge of the door. "Chris." She motioned to me with a sweep of her arm. "Next procedure is in the other room."

I had seen D&Es before and had assisted in a few. But I had never seen anything like what Rebecca had just done, in any surgical procedure. It wasn't like surgery at all, but like some athletic feat. She moved with the kind of speed and agility that made the whole thing look at once easy, beautiful, and also impossible. *Shit*, I thought. *I can't do that.*

A D&E is a more complicated and riskier procedure than a first-trimester abortion, mainly because of the greater blood supply to the uterus (higher risk of bleeding) and the use of forceps (higher risk of perforation). After removing the osmotic dilators, the doctor uses suction, as in a first-trimester procedure, to empty the bag of amniotic fluid, and to remove any smaller fetal parts that will pass through. Then, using forceps, she removes the remainder of the pregnancy. "Work your way up the fetus," Rebecca explained as

I watched the next procedure. "Start with the most proximal body part and then take the next, the next, the next. Calvarium, arms, trunk, legs, placenta. That's how to do a good D&E."

Rebecca's teaching, like her surgical technique, was efficient and methodical. On the third procedure, she had me remove the dilators, perform the bimanual exam and place the speculum. On the next procedure, she had me place the tenaculum—the instrument that grips the cervix to stabilize the uterus. On the next one, I used the cannula to break the amniotic sac.

I was clumsy and uncertain at first, using unfamiliar equipment and nervous under her gaze. Even though many of the steps were similar to those in a first-trimester abortion, I felt as though I were doing it all for the first time.

But Rebecca was patient and encouraging. She showed me how to hold the dilators from above and drop my wrist, pushing the angle of the dilator upward in order to "hug" the anterior wall of the cervix as I pushed through the internal os. She showed me how to work with my forceps in the lower uterine segment, feeling for something firm and confirming my position on the ultrasound, opening my hand wide and grasping whatever body part I could. She taught me how to make long, "directed" pulls with the cannula to dislodge any remaining tissue from the walls of the uterus. When I faltered, she stepped in, giving me pointers, making me watch her technique.

"See my hands? See my angle here? It's like a dance." And it was. She moved her body like a boxer or a ballerina—her stance wide, her arms strong, her movements precise and efficient. When she made her final pass with the cannula, she seemed to enter a quiet, internal space, like a pianist playing an exquisite chord progression: she closed her eyes, tilting her head slightly and tucking her chin. It was as though she were entering the small, invisible space inside the uterus and feeling her way around in the dark with her hands. Only she was doing it with a thin plastic cannula that was like an extension of her body, one long, sensitive finger.

With each patient, she had me add on a step, until I was doing the whole procedure myself. Early in the day, watching me use the forceps, she said, "You've got good hands, Chris. Good surgical hands." I grasped clumsily at the calvarium, feeling the roundness of it slip between my forceps. "That's okay. I can tell you're integrating what you're seeing on the ultrasound with what your hands are doing. Most family medicine doctors can't do that. That's excellent. Try again. Go on."

On the next procedure, I grasped the calvarium on the first try. "You've got really good hands," she said again. "I'm sure you've been told that before."

But no one had told me that before, or if they had, I didn't remember. I felt like I was flying, soaring under Rebecca's strong and beautiful wing.

In the mid-morning, in between cases, she picked up her phone and glanced at a text message, muttering to herself, "She's in pain? Why is she in pain?" Then looking up at me, she rolled her eyes. "My mom is such a drama queen. She's getting some veins removed from her leg today, and she's like, *Oh! Woe is me!* My sister is a totally non-medical person, but she's the one with our mom at the hospital. Because, you know," she gestured with both hands toward herself, "I'm here." She rolled her eyes again and tucked the phone in her pocket. "She's fine, she's totally fine. It's like a totally elective, minor surgery." I thought I heard a subtle tension in her voice—love, worry.

We returned to the procedure room.

"Did you bring lunch?" she asked me, after we'd done about twenty cases. "Bring it into my office. We'll talk."

I sat across from her. She gestured toward my leftovers with her chin. "Nice. You make that?"

I shook my head. "My friends did. Our dinner from last night."

"Nice," she said again. From her purse she removed a clear plastic box, a protein pack from Starbucks. "I can't even remember the last time I cooked. I eat, like, ten to twelve meals a week from Starbucks. So do my kids, actually."

She pulled out her phone and showed me a picture of two young girls. "My daughters," she said. "Five and seven."

"Adorable," I said. And they were. They had Rebecca's same olive skin, long eyelashes and dark, curly hair. They looked like happy children.

"You're married?" she asked, glancing at my ring finger.

I nodded.

"What does your husband do? Is he a doctor too?"

"Yeah, he is. An ophthalmologist," I said.

She nodded. "Okay. So he gets it, at least a little bit. What does he think about you doing this work?"

"He gets it," I said, using her words. "He does."

She chuckled. "That's good. That helps, I think. My husband doesn't have a clue. I mean, he knows what I do. But he's not a doctor. He's an industry guy. Music. He's kind of a germaphobe, actually. If he had any idea the stuff that gets all over me all day?

The stuff that splashes in my face? He wouldn't touch me."

I laughed. I liked her.

"I'm assuming you guys don't have kids?" she said.

I shook my head. "Not yet."

"But you want them?"

"Yeah," I said. "I do."

"They're the best thing in the whole world. The best thing. But who am I kidding? I don't have any time for them when I get home at the end of the day. Like, not even enough to say hi. Just, no." She held her hand up like a stop sign. "We belong to a twenty-four-hour daycare in downtown L.A. It's amazing. That's why I can do this. With the amount I work? It's insane. I know what you must be thinking: she can't keep this up forever. And I can't. I know it. This job is crazy. It's nuts."

"How long have you been doing it?"

"Since I finished fellowship," she said. "Two and a half years. And it's not slowing down. It's only speeding up. But whenever I complain about working too much, my husband says, 'Even if we had all the money in the world, you would keep working like this.' "

I chewed my lunch.

She shook her head again. "My daughter asked me to pack her a lunch the other day, and I was like,

'No, Honey. I'm not that kind of mom.'" She closed the empty Starbucks box and stuffed it in the trash. "But I hope they'll get it someday, you know? I hope they'll understand that I do important work, and I do meaningful work. And I'm just not that kind of mom."

We finished the day with a series of first-trimester procedures. After the tricky D&Es in the morning, I felt back in my element. Rebecca watched me closely on the challenging procedures, but during the routine ones she stood in the corner and chatted with the nurse anesthetist.

The last procedure of the day was a woman with an eight-week pregnancy and three prior C-sections. I was making my last pass with the 8-flex cannula, when suddenly I felt the fundus—the posterior wall of the uterus—disappear. I knew immediately what had happened. "Rebecca," I said, "I think I perforated."

She had been checking something on her phone. She looked up. "Suction off," she told the assistant. "Let me feel." She placed her hands on the cannula and probed the wall of the uterus, feeling what I did. "Yup, you did," she said. "You perforated." She didn't bat an eye. "Do you think you got everything out?"

"Yes, I think so," I said.

"Let's look," she said.

We took the suction container to the lab room and examined the contents. An eight-week size gestational sac floated in the Plexiglas dish. The abortion was complete.

We returned to the room. Rebecca felt around the walls of the uterus one more time, watching her movements closely on ultrasound. "Don't worry," she said. "She's going to be fine."

My face must have been ashen. "Have you ever perforated before?" she asked me.

"No."

She gave a little laugh. "The thing you have to remember is that abortions are one of the safest procedures there is. Perforation is like your worst nightmare, right? We're so careful to avoid it, and we should be. But now it's happened to you. You poked a little hole in her uterus. You have to watch her for bleeding, make sure you didn't suck any bowel through with your cannula. But ninety-nine percent of the time that doesn't happen. You'll watch her. She'll go home. This will heal itself up in a few days."

She handed me a copy of the clinic protocol for perforations, and told me to write the note detailing the procedure and my management plan. When the patient woke up, I told her what had happened and answered her questions. At the end of it, she was fine. She went home. We went home.

I couldn't wait to go back the next morning.

This is it, I told myself. *This is it.*

For the next two nights, I'd planned to stay with Mo's "cousin-brother" Aanand and his wife Charlene at their apartment in Beverly Hills. I'd visited them there before, but never without Mo.

Aanand was working long hours at his law firm. I didn't expect to see much of him, so I made all the plans with Charlene, who was a natural hostess. Charlene had told me she was also working that evening, although I wasn't entirely clear on what Charlene's job was. (I had heard her describe herself alternately as a "hustler" and an "artist.") So I knew I would have the apartment to myself that night, which was exactly what I wanted. Charlene left a key with the doorman.

The apartment was as always, immaculate and quirky: a red ceramic bull's head in the entryway with car keys dangling from its horns, a table lamp that looked like a glowing piece of rose crystal, a stack of style magazines under a skateboard wheel paperweight. Although I'd never seen any piece of art made by Charlene, whenever I walked into that apartment, I felt she had a right to call herself an artist. With her creative energy, her eye for aesthetic, and of course, her money, everything she touched became bright and important, impossible to ignore.

As I dropped my bag on the floor by the couch and pulled out my diary, it occurred to me that something about Charlene reminded me of Rebecca. They were certainly different from each other, and I was different from each of them. Yet I saw things in each of them that I wanted to emulate. They were both passionate people, and they didn't try to hide their passion or contain it. They were both the kind of people who could captivate a room—in an abortion clinic or in a penthouse apartment in Beverly Hills—with the energy that radiated from them.

That is what I want for myself, I thought. *I want to be like that.*

On the very first case the next morning, I perforated again. "Are you serious?" Rebecca said this time. But she wasn't angry.

"This is okay, this is good," she said, as we repeated the steps from yesterday: examining the products of conception, checking the patient's uterus with the ultrasound, drawing a hemoglobin level as she awoke in the recovery room. "You're learning from this. This happens."

But I was horrified. My hands shook as I started the next case.

"Drop your wrist," Rebecca said, watching me closely. "Directed pulls. Ease back up to the fundus. Good. Good, Chris."

Another case, then another. The speed of the day, the dance, began to come back. But I was the one who was keeping the rhythm now, not Rebecca. When I faltered or hesitated, she nudged me on. "Why are you still in the uterus? You're done. It's empty. Get out of there."

Next case. Next case.

At lunch, I asked Rebecca, "How's your mom doing? How did her surgery go?"

She laughed and rolled her eyes. "My mom," she said, picking up a hard-boiled egg from her Starbucks box, breaking it in half with her fingers. "She's fine. Her stupid leg veins. Jeeze. I was on the phone with my sister for like an hour last night. They're not medical people," she said again. "No one in my family is."

She asked me about my family. I told her about my dad. She listened. "How often do you see your dad?"

"Not very often," I said.

I told her about my writing.

"That's great," she said. "That's wonderful. So, after residency is over, you'll get to spend time with your dad. And you'll get to write again."

"That's my hope," I said.

She nodded eagerly, one hand to her mouth, chewing her egg. "You will," she said. "You'll do it. You're going to have so much time all of a sudden. You're not going to be like me. You're going to be balanced. And you'll have so many stories to tell." She raised her eyebrows. "Right?"

I thought about the night before, the hours I'd spent with my diary, thinking faster than I could write it all down: the clinic, the women, Rebecca's movements like a dancer, the feeling of the fundus disappearing under my cannula. "Yeah," I said. "A lot of stories."

The day went on. Another sixty abortions. Lots of stories.

We went home.

That night, Charlene took me out to dinner at a restaurant in Hollywood called Little Next Door. "My treat," she said. "I left you on your own last night, I'm gonna make it up to you." We sat in a garden strung with globe-shaped paper lanterns. The air smelled of jasmine and gardenia. We drank *kir royales* and white wine, shared heaping plates of mezze, then saffron pappardelle and sea scallops.

We talked nonstop, mostly about our husbands— "the Mehtani men," she called them—and their family.

For a long time we talked about Neil and about what happened to him, about the difficulties of his life: his vegetative father, passing the years in a fan-cooled room in India. The difficulty of being an immigrant—an overweight, foreign, brown-skinned teenager in an American high school. The fact of a mental illness never fully acknowledged, diagnosed, or treated. And there was something else, something I had thought about a thousand times but had never said out loud. There was the difficulty of being raised, supposedly like a son, in his uncle's home. But the truth is, he wasn't their son. His parents were far away, and they hadn't been there to save his life.

Maybe Neil's own parents couldn't have saved him, any more than his aunt and uncle could. But it was something I couldn't get out of my head. Where did the responsibilities of a parent begin and end? And could anyone, even family, take over where a parent left off?

It was a relief to speak these things out loud, and even more, to hear them spoken by someone else —another woman who, like me, could see into the depths of the Mehtani family, but who remained outside of it.

As I told Charlene about my difficulties trying to be a good doctor and a good wife, she said something about Mo that surprised me. I was telling her how, throughout residency, he had always wanted to do things together, even when I wanted nothing more than to be alone. She said, "He's co-dependent, like his parents."

"I guess so …" I thought for a moment. "But his dad's not really like that."

"Right," she said. "His dad is more like you and me: he does his own thing, he goes to work, he goes to the gym, he lives his life. It's Mohit's mom who is co-dependent. Mohit is like his mom."

Of course, she was right. I was so used to seeing all the ways in which Mo was like his father: his diligence, his work ethic, his gregarious social energy. It had never occurred to me that in this way, he was like his mother: the way he wanted to lean on me and intertwine his life with mine, the way he wanted me to lean on him. He was like his mother.

Over dessert, Charlene told me that she was trying to get pregnant.

"That's great," I said, cautious in my enthusiasm. Charlene was nearly forty; I thought her chances of conceiving might be slim, but I wasn't going to bring that up. Instead I asked, "How do you, ah, feel about the idea of motherhood?"

She rolled her eyes. "I don't know, it's going to be hard work. I've seen my sisters do it." She made a little face, picked up the bottle to refill our wine glasses. "I'm not going to be one of those moms that stays home all day and obsesses over her kid. No way. That shit isn't good for anyone. I already told Aanand if we're doing this, we're getting a live-in nanny."

I let out a little laugh, then caught myself, seeing that she was serious. "Okay. Great!"

"I want to keep working and living my life, you know?"

"Of course," I said. "You should."

Somehow of all people, I could see Charlene pulling it off: being a good mother, even if she didn't want to do the day-to-day work of it. Charlene was good at many things. She was good at being the person she was.

The next morning I was up early, restless with anticipation. My whole body ached from two days of back-to-back procedures. That night I would make the long drive home. One more day of abortions left. I couldn't wait to get back to the clinic.

I met Rebecca in her office. She waved me in.

"I think in all training," she said, between sips of coffee, "in your whole career in medicine, actually, your confidence kind of ebbs and flows like this"—she made a sine wave with her hand in the air. "You came in on the first day and you started to get really confident and comfortable by the end of the day. Then you had those perforations and your confidence kind of went down. Now it's coming back up. I think today you're going to hit your stride again. My goal is for you to peak in your confidence by the end of today."

I nodded. I started on the first case and did twenty-five procedures back-to-back.

She stood at my side and did nothing but watch and give tips here and there. "Drop your wrist. Hug the anterior wall." "Watch your tenaculum." "I like how you're making directed pulls. You're feeling for where the tissue is attached and you're targeting your tip there. That's good." Occasionally I would ask her to repeat my bimanual exam if the uterine orientation was tricky, or to confirm when I was pretty sure but not positive that the uterus was empty. But usually my intuition was right. "Yup, I totally agree with that exam. Very anteverted and anteflexed. Great." "You're right, there's just a tiny bit of something left at the fundus here. See if you can get it with one or two more passes. Good."

At lunchtime, she sent me home. "You've got a long drive ahead of you. You're not driving out of here on a Friday at 5 p.m. in traffic. Get going." She gave me a hug.

I pulled onto the freeway with my heart in my throat. It was exactly what I needed. Her hug, her reassurance. The whole trip. She was right: I did hit my peak. I'd found the thing I was good at, even gifted at. And finally, someone had shown me how it could fit into a whole life.

I thought about Rebecca's kids and their twenty-four-hour daycare. *They love it there.* I imagined Charlene as a mother, hiring a live-in nanny to stay with the baby while she was out "working." *I want to keep living my life, you know?*

I wasn't going to live Rebecca's life, or Charlene's life. But I respected the choices they were making, and the way they lived lives that felt complete and meaningful to them. *I do important work, meaningful work.*

The interstate slipped by me on either side, the pink and green of three days earlier already fading to summer brown, the blossoms blown away in the hot breeze. I drove in silence, listening to nothing but my own thoughts.

This is it. I was certain. *This is it.*

Rebecca offered me the job in Modesto, performing abortions one day a week. I graduated from residency and started working for her a few months later. I've been there nearly a year now. Soon after, I found a second job at a large Ob-gyn practice doing prenatal care and office gynecology. But the abortion work is still my love and my passion.

The Modesto clinic is a two-hour drive from our home: east through a hilly pass dotted with wind turbines, then south through the Central Valley. It is nothing like Rebecca's clinic in L.A. There are about half as many patients, for one thing, and less than a third of the staff. It's always busy, but nothing moves quickly.

It's a low-paying job, even for a young doctor straight out of residency. The place operates on a lean budget; most of the patients are on Medi-Cal, California's version of Medicaid. The building is clean, the staff is caring and conscientious. But there is no question that I'm in the trenches. Compared to the hospital-based clinic in medical school, where classical music played in the hallways and patients sipped green tea while recovering from anesthesia, the Modesto clinic is about as inviting as a dark bus station after midnight.

Plenty of doctors take pride in working in this type of setting, delivering no-frills medical care to the patients with the greatest need. I am not ashamed to work there. An abortion clinic doesn't need to look like a day spa. But the shabbiness of the place irks me. The outdated (albeit perfectly functional) equipment, musty old armchairs in the waiting room, the total absence of flowers on the desks or pictures on the walls—it all sends a message: *What do you need pretty pictures and flowers for? You're lucky someone is here to help you at all. So sit down and be quiet and wait your turn.*

And they do wait. In a large room lined with folding metal chairs, empty except for an old television mounted above the door, they wait for me for hours, sometimes all day. There are always so many women. And only one doctor.

The procedure room is a wide rectangle: white walls, linoleum floor, the smell of bleach and plastic. The exam table sits in the center of the room, upholstered in cracked vinyl. Two candy-cane hooks are attached to the far corners of the table, each with a wide loop of canvas dangling from it. Any woman, even one who has never been in a room like this, knows that those straps are where your feet go.

In a back corner stands an ancient mechanical ventilator, its cylinder stuffed with tiny nuggets like lawn fertilizer. A red cart with a dozen narrow drawers is topped with glass vials and a syringe. Beside the procedure table, a brown plastic box, about knee height, with metal handles on each side and two glass jars on top, connected by plastic tubing—the vacuum. Beside this, a bucket of water. A stool on four wheels—the doctor's chair.

There is no anesthetist, so the patients are sedated, but not asleep. This makes procedures more difficult, because I have to attend to the patient and keep her as comfortable as possible during a painful procedure. It is safer for the patient (general anesthesia is always riskier than a routine abortion procedure), and in truth, I prefer it this way. I like talking to the patients, keeping the whole woman in my mind even as I work through the narrow tunnel of the speculum.

There are a lot of things about this job that aren't quite what I expected, things that have begun to wear on me. It's not just about the shabby clinic or the line in the waiting room. (Unlike residency, at the end of the day, we always go home.) It has something to do with the patients. The things they say, the choices they make, the choices they don't get to make. The clarity is fading, the image warping, black and white blurring into each other. It is all beginning to seem more complicated than it did before.

One afternoon when I'd been working in Modesto less than a month, my very last procedure was a fifteen-week abortion in a G1P0—a woman pregnant for the first time.

It was about 5:30 and beginning to get dark outside. The clinic has no windows, but I was well aware of the time and of the long drive ahead of me. I walked through the swinging door into the procedure room and introduced myself to the woman on the table, who looked tired and somber. A few loose brown curls escaped from under the blue surgical cap the nurse had placed on her head. Her dark eyes looked straight into mine, but she hardly said anything, just nodded and gave one-word answers to my standard questions. She surely felt as I did: *I'll just be glad when this is over.*

It was a challenging case. The fetus felt larger than fifteen weeks—probably closer to sixteen, I thought. She hadn't had osmotic dilators placed the day before. Instead I had given her medications a few hours prior to the procedure to soften and open her cervix, but they'd barely had any effect. Her cervix was tight, the canal long and tortuous. I was working in a narrow space, and I was having a hard time maneuvering my instruments. The woman moaned in pain. As she writhed on the table, the ultrasound image kept moving; I had a hard time seeing my instruments on the screen. I kept telling Ronnie, the nurse, to give her more pain medication. But still she cried out with every move of my hands.

I know I am a young doctor. Sometimes procedures like this make me anxious. *Why is she in so much pain? Is there something wrong?* But I wasn't worried about those things that day. Everything seemed to be going smoothly, even though I could barely see what I was doing. That was fine. An abortion is a procedure done largely by feel, and this procedure, although it was difficult, felt normal. Except her pain, her moaning. Locking my teeth together, I told myself I had to keep going, let the nurse worry about her pain. My job was to complete the procedure safely.

When the uterus felt empty, I took the container back to the lab to inspect the products. Everything was there: the fluff of placenta, four tiny limbs, a spine and rib cage. But the calvarium, the easiest thing to leave behind, was missing. I would have to go back.

I returned to the procedure room. "I'm sorry," I told her. "It's not finished yet. I have to go in again."

"Okay, doctor," she said. Her head was turned to the side so I couldn't see her face. But I saw Ronnie reach over the table with a tissue to dab her eyes.

I placed the speculum again, washed her cervix, and held onto it tightly. I reached in with forceps and grasped, pulled. The woman let out a raw, open-throated cry. I looked down at my forceps: empty. I reached in again, grasped, pulled, felt some resistance, pulled harder, harder. Something loosened and emerged, coming through the cervix. There it was, crushed between my forceps, staring straight up at me: the calvarium.

"Got it," I said, and Ronnie and I both exhaled. It was over.

After packing up my things and changing my clothes, I went to the recovery room to see the patient. I asked her about her pain.

The cramps were still there, she said, but not as bad. She spoke perfect English with a thick Latin American accent. She thanked me profusely. I felt embarrassed and guilty. I had made her suffer.

Then she said, "You know why I did this?"

I shook my head.

"I didn't want to," she said. "But, you see, my husband died."

My breath caught in my throat. I took hold of her hand. "Oh, my dear. I'm so sorry."

She told me they had been together for nine years. They'd emigrated together from El Salvador, but they'd waited to have children, wanting to get settled and established in this country before starting a family. "Then this year, we decided to try. And I got pregnant right away.

"My husband, he is such a wonderful man. I loved him so much. But I can't do this without him. I didn't want to have the baby without him." Her voice was quiet and trembling, but it was also, in a way, hard, resolved.

"When did he die?" I asked.

"Last week," she said. "In a car accident."

Last week. Fifteen weeks pregnant. I glanced at her clinic ID bracelet: thirty-three years old. The same as me.

It is dangerous to identify too much with your patients, no matter what kind of doctor you are. Their problems are not the same as your problems, and it's vain and foolish to convince yourself otherwise. Nevertheless, sometimes you feel something, some link between your heart and hers, that is too powerful to brush aside.

I let go of her hand and brushed the tears as they rolled down her cheeks.

"Who is taking care of you?" I asked.

"My brother," she said.

"He's here with you today?"

"Yes."

Instinctively, I asked, "Do you have any sisters?"

She shook her head. No, it was just her and her brother. Their parents were killed at a young age. All the rest of their family was still in El Salvador, trying to stay alive.

I kept wiping her tears, stroking her hair, holding back my own tears. "You are a strong woman," I said. "I know this was a hard decision, even if you knew it was the right one. You need to just take care of yourself, now. Take time to grieve for your husband. Then you will go on and live your life."

"My life." Her voice echoed mine, and a faraway look came into her eyes. She gazed over my shoulder as though searching for something or someone she could not see.

When you're a resident, people are always telling you how to do things. Attending physicians like to point out differences in "style" or "preference," then they proceed to give you a detailed defense of why they do it this way or that way, as though it really were a matter of right and wrong.

But when you go out into the world and begin practicing on your own, you suddenly have the freedom—and terror—of choosing how you want to do things. Developing your own style.

A few of my teachers were more influential than others. My technical style mimics Rebecca's more than any of my other teachers. I hold the dilators the way she does, "hugging" the lower segment as I push through the cervix; I remove tissue through my cannula the way she taught me, using straight, "directed pulls" (I can still hear her voice in my head) rather than the spinning motion that many other doctors use. I still manage perforation according to the exact protocol we followed (twice) while I was training with her.

CHRISTINE HENNEBERG

But because my patients are almost always awake, the most important elements of my style lie in my words and demeanor. These things I learned from other family medicine doctors—TEACH trainers, mostly— and the nurse practitioner who trained me to place osmotic dilators as a medical student: *Never use the word "spread." Never push her legs open. Earn her trust.*

There are some things I do that I don't remember being taught. Someone must have taught me, or I came up with them on my own.

Before I start the procedure, I always ask the same three questions:

"Can you tell me your name and birthday?"

"What questions do you have for me?"

"Are you feeling sure of your decision?"

It was a cold day in January, back before I was pregnant. The patient was an African American woman, heavy-set, bundled in a sweater, a paper drape covering her naked hips. She was about fourteen weeks pregnant.

She answered me quickly and quietly, without meeting my eye. *No questions. Yes, I'm sure.*

I sat down between her legs. Ronnie stood at her shoulder. She gave her a small dose of sedative and narcotic, then nodded to me: Okay to begin.

Ronnie tried to make her usual gentle small talk, distracting the woman from fear or pain. As the medications kicked in, she began to relax, to open up. "I didn't want to be here today, you know," she told us. I remember her voice, heavy and soft under the medication. It was like a warm breath on that chilly morning, putting all of us at ease, even her.

Ronnie murmured, "It's okay. Nobody wants to end up here."

"But I just can't go through this time. I got kids already at home." From my secluded, light-filled perch between the woman's legs, I glanced up at Ronnie. A silent sigh passed between us. We both knew this was the best way to get a woman through these ten minutes: get her talking about the kids she already has.

Ronnie encouraged her. "Oh yeah?" she said. "How old are your kids?"

"Two and four," she said.

"Phew! You got your hands full, huh?"

"Yeah, I got two boys."

"Two little boys! Wow!" Ronnie was awed and admiring. Their voices drowned out the clink of metal at my fingertips.

"Uh huh. They a handful all right. And I been getting so sick. Every single morning I'm getting sick. That's how come I gotta do this, you know." Her voice was confident now, her inhibitions down, narcotic pulsing through her veins. Her knees were splayed wide, the flesh of her bottom sinking into the table. She was like warm dough in my hands. "I mean, we want more kids. But we want a girl this time. And when I got to be three months along and I was still getting sick every morning, my mama said, 'You know you gotta go in there to the clinic.'"

"Mm-hmm," Ronnie cooed to her. I kept my head bent low as I peered down the speculum.

"She said, 'You know you don't never get sick after three months if you havin' a girl.'"

I looked up. Ronnie's eyes were wide, glued to mine. She gasped, "Oh …"

My eyes fell again. I had just finished the dilation; a stream of clear fluid gushed from her vagina. In front of me, at the level of my heart, her cervix was wide open and gaping, soft and ragged like a sea anemone. There was nothing to be said or done. Suddenly, forcefully, I was the one without options—the doctor. Every choice, every freedom, I had yielded to her.

I felt as though the metal clinking between my hands was also locked around my wrists as I completed the procedure, finishing what I started. On the ultrasound screen, under a flurry of obscuring snow, I watched her fetus tumble under the tip of the cannula, somersaulting with every flick of my wrist, then disappearing from the cushioned warmth of her sacrum and whipping through my hands—gone. Her third little boy, or so she believed. This was her choice, but it was also mine. She was sure of her decision. I had to be sure, too.

Another day in Modesto, about halfway through the afternoon, I walked into the procedure room and met my next patient: a thirty-year-old woman who was already lying calmly on her back in her surgical gown, her feet flat on the table. Her hair was in neat braids and her nails were manicured. I introduced myself and started flipping through her chart. Glancing at the papers in my hands, she said, "So, it's not twins, right?"

"I don't think so," I said. "No one told me anything about twins. But let me take a look at the pictures." In this clinic, I reviewed the patient's entire medical history, including her ultrasound images, once she was already in the procedure room. The staff reviewed the chart with me in advance only if there was an abnormal lab value or another unusual finding—such as "multiple" pregnancies. I flipped to the crude black and white photo and squinted at it. The image was fuzzy but undeniable: two gestational sacs, each with a tiny fetal pole in the center. Next to the photo, Kat, the ultrasound technician, had printed the word "TWINS" in her neat handwriting.

I blew a frustrated breath between my lips. Someone had dropped the ball. This woman had gotten all the way back to the procedure room without anyone mentioning to me—or, apparently, to her—that she was carrying twins. (Later I learned that the ultrasound had been done two days prior, when no doctor was available to do the abortion, and that the communication breakdown had occurred when she was rescheduled for today's procedure.)

I apologized that no one had discussed the findings with her, and I told her that yes, the ultrasound showed two pregnancies side by side. Twins.

"Oh God," she said, her voice low and heavy. "Are you serious?" She pushed herself to a seated position, crossing her legs under her gown. "Then I'm going to have to talk to my husband."

She explained that she already had a set of twins at home, three-year-olds. They were delivered "three months early" because she had what sounded like a case of severe preeclampsia, or even eclampsia (seizures during delivery). "I almost had a stroke and died," she told me. "I was in intensive care for a week after they were born." The twins had serious medical problems as well, due to their extreme prematurity. "One of them just got her tracheostomy out last week. The other one still has hers." She asked Ronnie to bring her her phone, and she showed us a picture of two petite, smiling girls, their brown arms linked around each other, one with a tracheostomy collar around her skinny neck. I thought of all the strain, the worry, the expenses, everything she must have gone through over the past three years.

"If it's twins," she said, "then I can't do this today. We already talked about it, and my husband is very clear that if it's twins, then he doesn't feel right about me having a—you know, about this procedure."

I offered to repeat the ultrasound, to see if there were definitely two viable pregnancies, to give her the most current, accurate information with which to make a decision. "A lot can change in a couple days, especially with twins, especially this early," I said.

"Yes," she said, nodding. "Please look again." As I slipped the ultrasound probe inside of her, she called her husband on speakerphone and asked me to tell him what I saw. I spoke loud and clear, so they could both hear me. "There are two pregnancies," I said. "Both of them have a heartbeat. They are the same size, about six and a half weeks. Twins."

She didn't waver. She hung up the phone, thanked us, sat up and began gathering her things. Feeling somewhat panicked, I told her that with her history of severe preeclampsia and now a second twin pregnancy, she was at extremely high risk of getting preeclampsia again, and this time things could be worse. I also told her she still had plenty of time to think about her decision. "Technically you have up until twenty-four weeks," I said.

She made a face. "Oh no, I couldn't do it then, not at twenty-four weeks. No way."

I understood then that she was unlikely to change her mind. Her eyes were wide open. She wasn't convincing herself of anything. She was resigned.

After a long silence, while she kept gathering her things and I stood watching her, not knowing what to say, Ronnie broke in, beaming at her. "Well, congratulations to you! You're gonna have twins!"

I looked up. "Yes, congratulations!" But it sounded false on my lips. I knew Ronnie's impulse was correct: to say something positive and validating. It wasn't right of me to make this woman feel as though her pregnancy was a tragedy. My job was to support her in whatever choice she made. She was pregnant with twins; she deserved to be congratulated just like any other woman.

Still, the word "congratulations" sounded to me like a little too much, too soon. I didn't want to concede just yet. So I added, "Whatever you and your family decide to do, we'll be happy for you. We just want whatever is best for you."

Words are the most difficult and important thing. And the procedure itself, of course. Do no harm and all that. It's mostly easy to avoid harm with my instruments. Even mistakes—perforation, bleeding—can be fixed.

The importance of words is part of what drew me to this work. A pregnant woman needs a doctor who respects language, who will choose words carefully. Help her write a story that she can live with, even be proud of.

I still believe that. But like everything these days, it is getting more complicated.

The other day, there was a patient on the schedule for a seventeen-week abortion; she'd had six osmotic dilators placed the day before. But she didn't want the abortion anymore, one of the counselors told me. "She wants you to take the dilators out and leave the pregnancy inside."

I called her into my "office," a large, empty room with a computer and a few gurneys where patients sometimes slept while they waited for their procedures. She was in her late thirties, older than me. She wore a tight maroon tank top. Rolls of pale, doughy skin bulged from under the straps and around her armpits. A few tattoos lined her arms, her dark, damp hair was pulled back in a ponytail. "Tell me what's changed for you since yesterday," I said.

She explained that her husband had been in prison for over a year, and had gotten out on parole last week. In the meantime, she'd become involved with another man, and was now pregnant. Her husband had moved back in with her (he owned the house) and wanted her to end the pregnancy. So she'd come to the clinic yesterday to start the process.

She looked up at me, her jaw tight and determined. "But you know what? I got home last night with those things inside me, and something just didn't feel right. I don't just mean my belly cramping, I mean something emotional. I sat down and thought about it real hard, and I thought to hell with it. My husband, he's always coming and going, letting me down. Shoot, he'll be back in prison next year, I wouldn't be surprised. Then what?" She shook her head. "Naw. This time it's my decision. This is my baby, and I want to keep it."

I took a deep breath, treading carefully. "Yesterday," I said, "you signed some papers saying that you understood the risks of the procedure, including the risks of not coming back to finish it today."

"Right," she said. "I know. That's why I came back."

"I just want to be clear that the procedure—the abortion has already begun. When I take out those dilators, your water could break. Even if it doesn't, your cervix will stay open. That's dangerous for the baby, and for you. You could bleed. You could go into labor at any minute; the fetus would be too small to survive. You could get an infection in your uterus that would spread to the fetus. You could also die."

"I know that. I know. It's all on those forms. I read the forms."

"And you still want me to do this?" I asked.

"Look, like I said, I want to do everything possible to save my baby. If it doesn't work, it doesn't work. But at least I'll know I tried."

Not once did I use the word "baby" with her. This was one of the first principles of abortion care that I learned in medical school: It is a pregnancy, an embryo, a fetus. Not a baby. In this case, I probably could have said it. She may have even wanted me to say it. But I felt that it would be a lie.

I took her back to the procedure room and placed the ultrasound on her belly. "I'm just checking on the fluid first," I said, "and the heartbeat."

"Oh I know it's still alive," she said. "I can feel it moving."

And so I did what she'd asked me to do. I placed the speculum and found her cervix. The dilators peeked out at me like baby birds snuggled in a nest. I grasped one with small forceps, pulled gently. It came out easily. I grasped the next one, the next, the last. Her cervix gaped at me, wide and soft, but the amniotic sac didn't break. I removed the speculum. "Okay," I said.

"Done?"

"Yes."

She pulled her legs together. I checked one more time with the ultrasound.

"Can I see it?" she asked.

I turned the screen toward her. The fetus was curled in profile, its heart pounding at 150 beats per minute. A little hand seemed to flatten against the screen as though reaching for its mother. Suddenly she let out a sob of relief, so wrenching and surprising I felt my own eyes well up. She squeezed her eyes shut and the tears ran down her face. I reached for her hand. "Thank you, doctor," she said, looking up at me. "Thank you for saving my baby."

Sometimes there is no right thing to say or do. I never believed I was saving a baby. I believed this poor woman would (and by now I believe she probably did) experience a pre-term delivery of a non-viable fetus or, perhaps, a severely disabled infant. I made it clear that this was what I expected and feared for her. And she still made her decision. She still called it "my baby."

In a way, she reminded me of Toby, how overjoyed and open she was from the first moment, when her pregnancy was nothing but two points on a graph, a doubling of her hormone level. The way she named it before she'd even had an ultrasound, the way she talks about it every time I call. She calls it "her," calls it "Juniper."

Meanwhile I am thirty weeks pregnant and still keep the stroller and high chair in the garage, under a white sheet.

Now I wonder if I was wrong. Not in what I did for that woman, but in what I said. I think about the words she used, the words I used. I think she wanted me to call it that: her baby. But I wouldn't. It still makes me ache to think of it.

THIRTY-EIGHT WEEKS

WHEN I WAS A medical student on my obstetrics rotation, I worked with a doctor named Juan Vargas. Dr. Vargas is one of those doctors who is beloved by residents, students, and patients. He is one of the few obstetricians left in California who performs breech vaginal deliveries.

Almost all babies get themselves into a head-first position by thirty-six weeks: curled in a tight ball, ready for a smooth entry into the world. But a few—somewhere around three percent of all babies—will remain in a butt-first or "breech" position. These babies can still come out vaginally, but most obstetricians would prefer to avoid it. When the body comes out first, the head can theoretically get stuck inside, the jaw acting like a lever against the pelvic bones. "Head entrapment," they call it. At that point, it is too late to switch to a C-section. The baby is half in, half out. The cervix and vagina clamp down around the neck and the umbilical cord, cutting off the blood supply to the baby's brain. The baby dies.

As dramatic and horrible an outcome as this sounds, it is extremely rare. The only way to avoid it with certainty is to schedule the woman for a C-section before she goes into labor. But a C-section, though considered a "routine" surgery, is not risk-free either. It involves all the risks to the mother of a major abdominal surgery, plus some risks to the baby. So the decision of whether to deliver a breech baby vaginally or by C-section is not necessarily an obvious one—although these days, most obstetricians won't even offer a vaginal delivery to a woman whose baby is breech. They tell her that a C-section is recommended, and the discussion is closed.

Dr. Vargas wanted to make sure every woman with a breech baby had enough information to have a real discussion of her options, and to allow the woman to make the decision with her doctor. He asked me to review the literature and develop a concise, readable pamphlet, called a "decision-making aid," for women whose babies were breech.

Dr. Vargas was a good teacher. I think he knew I would learn more from this project than just the state of the medical research.

I did learn inside and out the true risks of breech vaginal delivery, which are extremely small. In the early 2000s, a large, rigorous study seemed to suggest that breech vaginal delivery was dangerous, compared to C-section. Very few babies died, but the babies born vaginally were more likely to have problems breathing after birth, low Apgar (neonatal well-being) scores, and longer hospital stays. When the researchers examined the two sets of babies several years later, however, they found that they were indistinguishable. Any of the problems present at birth in the babies born vaginally had been completely transient. No matter how they came into the world, for the most part all the breech babies grew into healthy children.

From this project, I also learned how to think about a nuanced and controversial topic in medical research and translate it into understandable language for the patient. This has proven to be an invaluable skill working in family planning.

Most importantly, I learned how hard it is for a pregnant woman to find a doctor who trusts her to make her own decisions about her pregnancy and birth. Everywhere a pregnant woman turns, she gets the same

CHRISTINE HENNEBERG

message: *You are not to be trusted with your own body.* It permeates every moment of the pregnancy, from the question of abortion to the final decision of how the baby will emerge from her body. It is a culture that pressures the woman to make decisions based on fear, rather than on reasoned discussions with her doctor or—heaven forbid—instinct and expertise in her own body.

I think about all the women who have said to me, "I have to check with my husband first." The ones who come in for an abortion, then change their minds after listening to their boyfriend or family or protestors outside the clinic. And the ones who, despite promising me that the abortion is their choice and theirs alone, have undoubtedly been pressured by a man, a parent, or some circumstance that I cannot begin to imagine.

The baby is breech. I've started calling it that now: the baby. Because everyone else does, even strangers, people in the grocery store. At this point, no matter how it comes out, I suppose it will be a baby. My baby.

I've tried everything: yoga, acupuncture, ice packs, hand-stands in the pool. Every night, Mo lights a moxibustion stick and swirls it around my little toe, then lies next to me on the couch while I try to imagine the baby flipping somersaults inside of me. Dr. Fineberg, my obstetrician, tried three times to turn it, pushing on my belly with her hands, but she gave up. "This baby doesn't want to move," she said. "I don't want to hurt you."

Everyone tells me to just have the C-section. I printed out all the studies for Mo, and he read them carefully. He didn't read the books I gave him about natural childbirth or mindful parenting, but he read the medical studies. I even gave him the pamphlet I wrote as a medical student. And still he says he thinks the answer is obvious: the safest thing is to have a C-section.

But it's not obvious to me.

Dr. Fineberg is like Dr. Vargas. She has made a practice of trusting women. She is experienced at this, she delivers breech babies regularly, and she has told me she will try to deliver it vaginally if that's what I want. "You know the data as well as I do," she says.

Yes, I keep thinking, and I know something even better: I know my body. I know my gut. And I trust it.

This is what I want. I don't want to bypass a natural process. I don't want someone to take a scalpel to my abdomen and yank my baby out of me like a melon from a grocery bag. I don't want to make a decision based on fear.

Even though I am terrified. Of course I am.

I've started seeing an acupuncturist in town named Irit. She does me a lot of good. She doesn't just stick the needles in me and promise me she'll make the baby flip. She is more honest than that. She asks me about my fears about the pregnancy, about motherhood, about the baby. I told her I'm afraid the baby will die.

Irit said, "You've seen too much. The story of this birth and this baby have been taken away from you—by your work, by your knowledge, by all the things you've seen. Now it's time to take it back. You get to be a mother now. You get to rewrite the story."

Twice a week I go to her office, where there is the smell of burnt herbs and the sounds of waves crashing and the warm glow of the lamps. She has me lie on the table and close my eyes and imagine the birth. "Rewrite the story," she says. "How does it end?"

FORTY WEEKS

A WILD GOOSE FLIES south for its first winter, following a compass written in its genes. A high school French teacher makes her first pilgrimage to Paris the summer after she retires. A priest dies and enters heaven. Is it what they imagined?

How do you go to a place you know about, a place you never doubted, a place you've described a thousand times but have never seen?

In the dark middle-of-the-night, alone in the house, what I felt was at once familiar and unknown to me. It was a sensation I had described to thousands of women, with a confidence ("fake it till you make it") inherited from generations of residents before me, men and women who had never experienced labor contractions but had to tell their patients what to expect. *A tightening in your whole belly. Intense. Painful. It will feel different from anything you've felt before.* Validating, in a way, to recognize the very thing I had heard myself describe so many times. *Not bad, Chrissy. Not too far off, after all.*

There was very little buildup to the contractions. They came strong, and they came relentlessly. When I couldn't stay in bed any longer, not wanting to wake Mo, I put on my slippers and sweater and shuffled out into the cold night. For what seemed like hours I walked back and forth on the length of our street, in this known world of Christmas lights and frosted lawns and the glowing orb of the moon in the sky. With each contraction I had to stop, grabbing on to whatever I could: a fence, a mailbox. *You'll know they are true labor contractions*—my own words now echoing in my head and in every cell in my body—*because you can't walk or talk through them.*

I did not think about the breech, the fact that this baby was coming out bottom first. Only that it was coming.

In the shower, the water moving over my body seemed at once to be inside of me and also outside of me, holding me, carrying me like a river.

At about 2 a.m. I decided to wake up Mo. He didn't seem to understand what I was telling him at first, but when the next one came and he saw me bend over and moan like a barn animal, he understood.

"I've never hit every single green light before," he said happily as we zipped through town. Our friend Parie, a nurse midwife who I'd originally hoped would deliver the baby, drove behind us. For a while I just lay in the backseat on my side, but when the contractions picked up again on the highway, I rose onto my hands and knees, rocking back and forth and noticing the low, round moon watching me from the safety of the black sky.

All Labor & Delivery wards are basically the same: a hallway lined with poster-sized photos of sleeping babies or mothers with silk sheets draped over their shoulders, the dome of a milk-full breast rising over the fold. Heavy wooden doors leading to rooms with drawn curtains, a wide bed in the center. Across the bed a set of two blue straps, fetal monitors, wait to be wrapped around the woman's gravid abdomen for constant data collection, like an astronaut in outer space. A computer screen and a row of wall hookups that can be attached to life-saving streams of oxygen, fluids, blood.

At the end of the hallway, a wide metal sink next to a set of swinging metal doors, each with a tiny rectangular window: the operating room.

Because of Kaitlyn's baby, because of (as Irit said) the things I have seen, I did not want to have this baby in the hospital. But because of the breech, it was the only safe way.

The nurse who checked me in called me "Dr. Henneberg" and asked if I had any preferences or requests. After the contraction passed I told her I preferred to be called "Chrissy," and I requested to be treated like a patient and nothing else, like I didn't know this place or these customs, like I had never been here or anywhere like it before.

Then there were hours. The contractions were nothing but a game of endurance and positioning. Surviving each one, not thinking about the next. Mo's hands were on my back. Parie encouraged my movements and my sounds, low, guttural moans that felt like they came straight from my belly. Dr. Fineberg told me the baby was safe and the heartbeat was excellent; I did not look at the monitor because I did not want to interpret the tracing myself.

During one particularly awful contraction, I heard Parie say, "You're almost through this one, Chris. Another thirty seconds and it'll be over. Thirty seconds! You can do anything for thirty seconds." I thought of residency, and in my mind I answered: *I can do anything for three years.*

I lost my taste for water and food, but at one point when I was bent over the edge of the bed, leaning on my arms, my hips rocking in the air behind me, Parie placed a paper towel on the bed in front of me. Upon it was a slice of orange, peeled and cold. She offered it to me, and I let her place it in my mouth, the cold membrane on my tongue and the burst of its juice like a gift, the sweetest thing I ever tasted. I ate another slice, and another.

A short time later, I threw them all up. Then they told me my cervix was open. It was time.

"Push!" they said.

But there was nothing, no space to push into, only pain and a dead end.

How many times had I said that word—"Push!"— to a woman in labor? And yet the word had no meaning to me now. That was the worst part. This place that was like the Paris of the schoolteacher and the heaven of the holy man; this direction that was like the true north of the geese—this was supposed to be my place. But it turned out to be nowhere. The words I knew turned out to have no meaning, like a language learned from books, failing me in this foreign place. I had no map or compass inside of me. I had no knowledge or intuition of how to do this last and most important thing.

They moved me into the operating room as a precaution, the bed banging through the swinging metal doors. Suddenly there were more people and many wires attached to me. Still I was trying to find direction and strength, a place I could push into. But every time I moved I became more tangled, the wires wrapped around my wrists, my arms, my belly. And I thought, *What if I can't do this?*

The only evidence of the breech was the dark meconium that began to ooze out of me. "I'm pooping!" I said. "No," said Parie, "that's the baby's poop." Gradually I understood that my contracting uterus was squeezing this stuff out of the baby's intestines, out of its body and onto the delivery bed— that's how close it was. I was coated in it, sliding in dark grease like those wild birds after an oil spill, their feathers slick and black, their frowning beaks and their wet eyes begging: *Help.*

Dr. Fineberg pressed her hand inside of me, spreading her fingers, as she tried to give me direction and encouragement. She was saying the same things I'd said a thousand times to so many women in labor. *Push against my fingers! Push right into my fingers!*

But even though I knew exactly what she was telling me to do, I couldn't feel it, couldn't respond to it. All I could feel was the pain. "Please, stop!" I said.

The nurses kept trying to turn me onto my side, but that was where the pain was the worst. I kept begging them, "No! Please! I don't like it there!"

Then Dr. Fineberg's voice rose above everything else, suddenly stern: "I know you don't like it, but your baby likes it. You need to do it for your baby." I heard the change in her voice, and I recognized what it meant. The nurse leaned down and said to me, almost in a whisper, that the baby's heart rate had dropped. It had been below ninety for two minutes, and now it was time for the baby to come out.

"Do you understand what we're saying, Chrissy?" she asked me.

"They want to do a C-section," I said, as though I were a resident watching the case.

"Yes. Is that okay with you?"

"Yes, that's fine. Just do it. Whatever you need to do."

The nurse had done what I asked her not to do, she had told me something that only a doctor would understand—but it was what I needed. I knew what a heart rate below ninety meant: it meant a blue baby, a baby that didn't have much time left, a baby that needed to come out now. How quickly I was resigned to it.

The anesthesiologist called for his medications, and they moved me from the wide delivery bed to the narrow OR table. I somehow thought that everything would stop in that moment: the contractions, the pain, the chaos. I had the distinct thought that they would have to put me under general anesthesia and that in a few seconds this would all be over, and then I would wake up and see my baby.

But that was before the next contraction came, a contraction unlike any of the others because it brought something with it: that "urge." The "urge to push" that everyone talks about. Now I felt it.

But it was not a "push"—that wasn't the word for it. Of course. It wasn't my fault for not feeling what I was supposed to. It was the fault of the language. It's the wrong word. All of us have been shouting at women to "push!" for hundreds of years, and that's not what we really mean at all. What I felt was an involuntary heaving, like vomiting up those orange slices a few hours earlier. Only this heaving did not come from my stomach. It was in the bones of my pelvis, my abdomen, my whole body. To push suggests a bearing down or a contracting of space to create pressure. What I needed to do was open: to wait for that urge from my body, its signal of wanting to expel something, and then to put all my mental and physical energy into opening the bones and sphincters and bands of my pelvis, against every ounce of fear and pain that was searing through those places, and allow that urgent, expellant force to work and move the baby through me. It was not that I didn't have to do any work—I did. But "push" is not the word for it. "Open" is the word for it.

On my hands and knees on that narrow OR table, tangled in wires and smeared with meconium, I resolved, like every woman before me, to get my baby out. I let those urges swallow me whole. I opened.

I felt the tremendous, burning pain inside my vagina that I knew was what they called "the ring of fire." I knew then that I had gotten the baby where it needed to be and it was coming out of me. After one great urge and opening, I heard someone say, "Body is out, head is still inside."

So there it was: my baby. Dangling by its neck from my vagina.

Probably they yelled at me then to "Push!" again. But I wasn't listening. I knew that this was the end of the story, the moment when either I would have a baby or I would have nothing. And with the next contraction, it was almost ... easy. I opened again. Probably it was painful, but more than the pain I was focused on the movement: the sensation of it happening, the speed and the elemental transformation of it. I felt it come out of me, the head, and then I felt an instant closure and emptiness in my pelvis and my vagina, the sealing shut of a potential space.

Then a calm voice told me, "Chrissy, you're not going to hear her crying, because she's not breathing."

It was like I had been knocked down by a wave into a churning ocean. I did not know up from down, light from dark. There was only the roaring silence in my ears and an absence of time or space. I remember searching for Mo's voice or face, asking him, "Why isn't she breathing? Is she okay? Is she okay?" And Mo leaned over me and told me he didn't know, he wasn't looking at her, he was afraid to look. The nurses had her, someone said, and they were breathing for her with a bag. It might have been a few seconds or a few minutes that passed in that silent ocean, when I didn't know what I had: Did I have a baby, or did I have nothing?

Then someone said, "Dad, come over here! Come see your baby girl!" And right then I heard a little gurgly yelp, and then a wail. It was her.

And for that instant, everything else slipped away, all the boundaries and bodies in the world dissolved. There was no me or her, there was no us. There was just that cry, that voice, that breath, and it was the whole sky and the whole world.

They slid her up on the table so she was below me. I was crouching over her on my hands and knees, and I could see her: this squirming, blood-smeared human being, my baby, still tethered to me by her white, pulsing cord. I let my head drop between my arms and covered her with my whole self.

She was here. My baby. My baby.

This was the only thing I wanted, and now I had it. When Irit told me to "rewrite the story," this was the ending I wrote.

Some stories do have an ending: I gave birth to my baby girl. In the wide world of mothers and babies and birth, even with the breech, it was a smooth birth, uneventful. But for me, of course, her birth was the climax to a story I would tell over and over, to anyone who asked.

We called our parents and sisters that afternoon from the warm glow of our hospital room.

"Mom, you're crying," I said, when I heard her choked voice.

"Oh Chrissy … a girl!"

I gave a little laugh. "Is that what you wanted?"

"Well, I just … I just think every woman deserves a little girl."

Mo's parents came to the hospital. His mom brought Ziploc bags stuffed with a traditional mixture of ground nuts, fruits, and grains meant to fortify me and my breast milk. She cupped my face in her hands, her thumbs touching the outer corners of my eyes. In her gaze and her touch, which were filled with the purest love and relief, I understood something I hadn't before. I felt, and still feel, swirling in the ocean of my happiness and good fortune, a thin, cold current of shame: for all my judgments and misinterpretations, for the safety I'd taken for granted. "You have done it," she said. "You worked very hard."

That evening we texted a few friends. Toby responded immediately, ecstatic.

!!!!!!!
CHRISSY CHRISSY CHRISSY!
I AM SOOOOOO HAPPY FOR YOU! JUNIPER
AND I ARE JUMPING FOR JOY!
I CAN'T WAIT TO MEET HER!!!!
I AM SENDING SO MUCH LOVE TO YOU
THROUGH THIS PHONE RIGHT NOW!!!!
<3 <3 <3 <3 <3 <3 <3

We went home with our baby.

A few days later, I got another text message from Toby:

Chrissy, I have sad news.

The day of my daughter's birth, a few hours after Toby and I texted each other, Toby went into labor. She was eighteen weeks pregnant.

She didn't realize what it was. She thought it was something she'd eaten, maybe a stomach bug. She stayed up all night, rocking on her hands and knees on the living room floor. In the morning they drove to the ER, where a resident performed an ultrasound—saying nothing, not looking Toby or Kersh in the eye—and stepped out to call an attending.

Within an hour the baby was on the table between her legs.

I know what those babies look like: pink, translucent, big skulls and little salamander bodies. But that's not how Toby described it. "She was beautiful," she told me. "She looked like me, Chrissy. She was beautiful and perfect and tiny, but she was too tiny to live."

She would tell me this story over and over, on the phone, those first few days. All the while I was nursing my daughter, trying to keep her from cooing or crying whenever she came off my nipple. But I couldn't hide anything from Toby. "What are you doing right now?" she would ask me. "Are you nursing her?"

"Yes," I told her guiltily. "I am."

She would call me every day from her rocking chair, where she was looking out over the ocean, expressing her breast milk by hand. "The doctor told me I shouldn't do it, or my milk will never dry up. But that's the point. I don't want it to dry up."

She would tell me about the things she was feeling in her body: her bleeding, her soft, flaccid belly, her yearning—a physical need—for her daughter. "I bet our bodies are going through a lot of the same things right now, the same changes in the hormones and stuff." Her voice was soft, far away. "Do you think that's true?"

"Well, yes, in some ways," I said.

"But the difference is that you're holding your beautiful healthy baby in your arms. And my baby Juniper is gone."

What can you say to someone grieving like that?

The truth is that I was in a state of pure bliss. I loved my daughter with the ecstatic joy that only a new mother can feel. All the things people say about that kind of joy, I felt all of it.

After we hung up, I cried for Toby and her lost child, her baby Juniper. But I cried most of all out of relief—the feeling, the knowledge, that I had been skipped. The thing I'd believed would happen to me had happened to Toby instead. It happened within hours of my and my daughter's deliverance, of our slipping through the gates, passing into safety.

Some things happen, and some things just don't. The gates swing open, or they are slammed shut—by the hand of a doctor, a court, a choice. Or by no one, for no reason at all.

I could hear the clang ringing in my ears, vibrating in my bones. I turned back to my baby. I felt the warm, solid weight of her on my chest. She let out a shuddering breath. She slept.

EPILOGUE

YESTERDAY AT THE CLINIC, a protestor watched me from the sidewalk as I pulled into the parking lot. I felt his eyes on me as I got out and opened the trunk for my bag. We keep a stroller in the trunk, like any other parents of an eight-month-old.

Oh, look at that! he yelled at me across the lot, the vitriol in his voice coating me like grease. *That's hypocrisy if I ever saw it. The baby killer has a stroller in her trunk. How do you live with yourself? Killing babies in the morning and go home in the evening and put the baby in the stroller. You are sick!*

I closed the trunk, holding back tears. I walked to the door of the clinic.

He called after me. *Repent! Repent, baby killer!*

How do I continue to do this?

The answer is that most of the time I see and feel no connection between my work in the abortion clinic and my work as a mother. Most of my colleagues are mothers—I am not some aberration. My patients are also mothers. I don't mean this in a tragic sense, that they are mothers to some "unborn children" as the protester on the sidewalk would have you believe. They are mothers like me, in every sense: they live in a world without clear boundaries, because the moment you become a mother, the moment another heartbeat flickers inside of you, all boundaries fall away. They are mothers who must make choices and live with the choices that aren't theirs to make—because there is no other way to be a mother.

But the mind plays games with you. Anyone who has known the delicate curl of her own baby's fingers and toes knows what I'm talking about. You feel that tug inside you. For most women, it happens at the grocery store, or when they're out for a walk on a sunny afternoon. They see a young mother walking with a stroller (me) and they exclaim, "Oh, look at those cute, wiggly little toes!"

For me, this happens at the clinic, in the lab with my tweezers and my clear plastic dish. When I see those little fingers and toes, especially at the gestational age of eighteen weeks or so, I feel that tug. I think of my baby. I think of Toby's baby Juniper.

But I must also remind myself that this is not a baby. This was a pregnancy, and it is over. My patient is in the next room, lying on the table with a heating pad pressed to her belly while she waits for me to come back in and tell her that she can leave.

I say the same thing every time: "The abortion is over. You're not pregnant anymore. Nothing about the procedure will affect your ability to get pregnant in the future."

My daughter is with me everywhere these days, not just at the abortion clinic. When I sit in my shed and write, I keep my iPhone face up on my desk, the baby monitor app alerting me to her every slumbering movement, every breath and shuddering sigh. The sound of her white noise machine—a static buzz meant to sound like rainfall—permeates the silence of my thoughts, the click of my fingers on the keyboard. When she awakens and cries, her voice calls me back from wherever I am on the page, and I go to her, leaving a part of myself behind until the next time I can return to it.

It is a different life, in many ways. And in many ways, it is the same. I am the same woman, sitting here writing this, as I was when I circled the fire with Mo on our wedding day and when I wandered the hospital hallways as an intern. My hopes and dreams for myself are the same now as they were then. I am a doctor, a writer, a wife, and now a mother. Contrary to all my fears, becoming a mother has not made me any less of what I was. It has somehow made me more of it.

In the first few months after residency ended, before Mo and I started "trying" and were just *being*, I used to ask him, "Do you think things are better? Do you feel more loved?"

He would say, "Yes"—not very convincingly. Once he simply said, "I guess so," and it crushed me. But I can see now that it all felt just as tentative and uncertain to him as it did to me. Neither of us knew whether "better" was something we could trust, or even how to measure it. This has taken time.

Of all the things that make us more confident and secure in our marriage now, I think it is the fact that we have a child together.

Some things haven't changed. My dad still struggles against the trap of his frail body. My mom still follows him around the house, trying to keep him from knocking into something, falling, dying.

We still barely speak of Neil. Mo and I talk about him sometimes, alone. But his parents—I hardly ever hear them say his name. I know it's not because they don't think of him. Having a child of my own has helped me to understand fear and silence in a way I didn't before. Some things we view through a veil or a sieve because we don't want to see the whole picture. Some things we cover with a white sheet because we can't bear to look underneath. Some things are too great to speak of.

If there is one thing my work has taught me, it is this: there are no boundaries, really. We make our own, or at least I do. We try to keep things neat and acceptable. But in reality, everything is messy. The work of doctors, the bonds of family, the love of husbands and wives, mothers and children.

And yet somebody has to do the work, all of it: the work we love, and the work we hate. The work we are not particularly good at. We have to make choices, and we must live with the things that were never ours to choose. The things that happen, and the things that don't.

Toby is pregnant again. Another XX chromosome embryo implanted and is growing inside of her. Another baby girl, she tells me.

When Toby and I talk on the phone on these cool evenings that are turning once again toward fall,

I know she is sitting in her rocking chair looking out over the ocean, waiting for the day when she will bring her baby home and hold her in her arms. She calls her by her name, Sage. And so do I. "Toby," I say, "your baby Sage loves you. She can hear your voice, and she is waiting to meet you. And she loves you very much."

ACKNOWLEDGMENTS

I am grateful to the family members, friends, mentors, and colleagues who read and advised me on the manuscript. Thanks to Flip Brophy, Caroline Michel, John McMurtrie, Brooks Becker and Sarah Lahay.

I am particularly thankful to my husband, Mo, for supporting me throughout the writing and publishing process. Above all, I am indebted to all the mothers who appear in this book.

ABOUT THE AUTHOR

CHRISTINE HENNEBERG is a writer and a practicing physician. She earned a BA in English/Creative Writing from Pomona College and an MD and MS in health and medical sciences from the UC Berkeley — UCSF Joint Medical Program. She lives in California. *Boundless* is her first book.

9 798986 066707